HEALTH, HEDONISM AND HYPOCHONDRIA

HEALTH, HEDONISM AND HYPOCHONDRIA

The Hidden History of Spas

Ian Bradley

TAURIS PARKE
Bloomsbury Publishing Plc
50 Bedford Square, London, WC1B 3DP, UK
1385 Broadway, 5th Floor, New York, NY 10018

BLOOMSBURY, TAURIS PARKE and the Diana logo are
trademarks of Bloomsbury Publishing Plc

First published in Great Britain in 2020

A catalogue record for this book is available from the British Library
Library of Congress Cataloguing-in-Publication data has been applied for

ISBN: HB: 978-0-7556-2646-5; eBook: 978-0-7556-2666-3

2 4 6 8 10 9 7 5 3 1

Typeset in Adobe Garamond Pro by Deanta Global Publishing Services, Chennai, India
Printed and bound in Great Britain by CPI (UK) Ltd, Croydon CR0 4YY

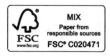

To find out more about our authors and books visit www.bloomsbury.com
and sign up for our newsletters

CONTENTS

ACKNOWLEDGEMENTS

This is a book that I have been thinking about and effectively working on for around forty-five years. Over that time, I have had considerable assistance in my travels and research in spas across Europe. Some of the names of those who helped me in earlier years are mentioned in this book but others, I fear, are now forgotten. Nick and Jane Ostler, James and Jane Bradby, and Stephen and Rosie Shipley have provided hospitality during research trips to Bath and Buxton, and Stephen and Alice Bates entertained me in Tunbridge Wells. More recently, I have benefited from meeting and speaking to Gaëtan Plein in Spa, Petra Nocker and Elisabeth Scharf-Kuen in Bad Wörishofen, Hans-Jürgen Sarholz in Bad Ems, Kurt Zubler in Baden bei Zürich and Stephan Wagner, Anita Basu, Matthias Fenzl and Irina Taculina in Bad Ragaz. Marianne Kusterer and Luana Wüstiner arranged a fascinating programme for me during my time at the Grand Resort, Bad Ragaz, and Denise Kirchner-Caminada gave me a thrilling tour of the Tamina Gorge. Carl and Helen Smith of Operetta Heaven have made my many visits to Bad Ischl and Baden bei Wien even more pleasurable experiences than they would otherwise have been.

I am very grateful to Benjamin Morgan for permission to quote from his PhD thesis on 'The Continental Spa in Post-1840 British, Russian and American Writing'. Jayne Parsons, Claire Browne and Natasha Collin at Bloomsbury have been unfailingly encouraging and supportive and Patrick Taylor was an exemplary copy editor.

As always, my chief debt is to my wife, Lucy, who has put up with my obsession with spas over four decades with patience, forbearance and a certain amount of wry amusement.

INTRODUCTION – *DER KURSCHATTEN*

A spa nowadays can be anything from a hot tub in the back garden to an exotic beach resort offering mindfulness and ayurvedic yoga. The word is regularly used by nail bars, hairdressers and other outposts of the booming beauty and wellness industry that seem ever to expand as most other high street businesses are contracting. According to figures produced by the Global Wellness Institute in 2018, new spas are opening around the world at a rate of 8,000 a year and there are now over 150,000 'spa locations' employing 2.6 million people and contributing $120 billion annually to the $4.2 trillion global wellness economy. Thermal and mineral springs, counted as a separate category, employ a further 1.8 million and generate $56.2 million annually.

The 2010 Global Spa Summit defined spas as 'establishments that promote wellness through the provision of therapeutic and other professional services aimed at renewing the body, mind and spirit'. Historically, the term has much more specific connotations. First adopted in the early fourteenth century by the resort based around natural mineral springs in the wooded hills of the Ardennes, near Liège in what is now Belgium, which still bears the name Spa, there are conflicting theories as to its etymology. Some maintain that it derived from the Walloon word *espa*, meaning fountain, others that it was an acronym of the Latin phrase *sanitas per aquam*, attributed to the emperor Nero. It is more likely to come from the Latin verb *spargere*, meaning to sprinkle or moisten, and specifically from *sparsa fontana* (a gushing fountain). The word was brought into wider currency by two English doctors who visited the original Spa in the early seventeenth century and came to be applied, initially in the

English-speaking world but later more generally, to all those places possessing natural springs, rich in minerals and often coming out of the ground hot or warm, to which people resorted to drink or bathe for therapeutic purposes.

These specific connotations are clear in the various names that have been applied to spa resorts across Continental Europe – *villes d'eaux* or *stations thermales* in French, *Heilbäder* or *Kurorte* in German, *terme* in Italian, *balnearios* in Spanish, *lázně* in Czech, *gyógyfürdők* in Hungarian, *banjas* in Serbo-Croat and *zdroje* in Polish. In North America the preferred term has been 'springs'. These words emphasise the presence of thermal water and the practice of bathing. Continental Europeans have tended to think in terms of 'taking a cure', as indicated by the French and German terms for spa-goers, *curistes* and *Kurgäste*, rather than use the English phrase 'taking the waters'. But all are agreed on the importance of the waters to spas and their properties have been the subject of much analysis and precise definition. Thermal mineral water is recognised as such when its temperature at source exceeds 20 degrees Celsius (68 degrees Fahrenheit) and/or its mineral content is at least one gram of dissolved salts or solids per litre or kilogram of water.

This book is about the historic, traditional spas of Europe. They include such well-known resorts as the original Spa in Belgium; Bath, Buxton and Harrogate in Britain; Baden-Baden, Bad Ems and Wiesbaden in Germany; Vichy and Aix-les-Bains in France; Baden bei Zürich and Bad Ragaz in Switzerland; Bad Ischl and Baden bei Wien in Austria; and Marienbad and Karlsbad in the Czech Republic. Those located in Continental Europe are still for the most part thriving as spas, unlike those in Britain, where sea bathing took over from inland spa cures and the coming of the National Health Service sounded the death knell for spa medicine. Occasional mention will also be made of those transatlantic offspring of the European spas, the White Sulphur Springs of Western Virginia and Saratoga Springs in Upstate New York.

These spas were the pioneers of the vast modern wellness industry and are now part of it, providing natural therapies and remedies as an alternative to conventional drug-based, high-tech medicine. They continue to offer, as they always have, escape, distraction and diversion, especially for the well-off and the stressed, and to pander to the eternal search for the body beautiful and the desire to cheat age and decay. They stand in a long tradition. The therapeutic benefits and pleasures of bathing in thermal mineral waters were first seriously appreciated by the ancient Greeks and Romans, who developed a rich social culture based around communal baths. After a somewhat fallow period in the Middle Ages, spas came into their own again in the sixteenth century thanks to serious scientific analysis of their waters by members of the new medical profession. They began to attract royal and aristocratic patronage and to develop cures for a huge variety of ailments and conditions based on taking their waters both internally and externally. Many in the upper and increasingly also in the middle classes took themselves off to a spa for 'the season' – usually the summer months – to escape the overpowering heat, stench, noise and general unpleasantness of city life and recharge their batteries. They were in many ways the earliest vacationers or holiday-makers. Spas established themselves as the first holiday resorts, adding luxury hotels, assembly rooms, theatres, concert halls, casinos and other places of entertainment to their core health facilities of bath houses and pump rooms or drinking halls.

In their heyday, from the mid-eighteenth to the early twentieth centuries, Europe's spas were the main meeting places for royalty, aristocracy and political, business and cultural elites; centres of political and diplomatic intrigue; and fertile sources of artistic, literary and musical inspiration and creativity. They became known as the cafés of Europe, a phrase first applied to Spa and Baden bei Wien. They epitomised style, luxury and ostentation and were renowned for their cosmopolitan atmosphere and glittering whirl of balls, gambling and flirtatious assignations as much as for their healing waters.

The history of spas can be approached from several different angles – medically and scientifically, by analysing their waters, their claims and their cures; architecturally, by looking at their distinctive buildings based around a landscaped *Kurpark*; politically, by charting their significant role in major events in European history; culturally, by exploring their influence on literature, music and art; spiritually, by probing their origins in religious cults based around water and medieval holy wells and their appeal as places of pilgrimage; sociologically and anthropologically, by analysing their distinctive clienteles, the motives that took people there and the distinctive spa 'types'; and from a business and economic perspective, by examining their development as the first true holiday destinations and pioneers of the tourism and travel industry. There is a rich range of literary sources on which to draw in the numerous travel diaries, novels, poems and letters written in and about them.

This book uses several of these different approaches and many of these sources to look below the surface and probe the more hidden aspects of the history of spas and what might be described as their secret or shadow side. It follows on from my earlier studies of the relationship between spas and music-making (Bradley 2010) and the place of spas in the wider spiritual history of water (Bradley 2012).

Spas are often hidden places in a very literal sense, sited in remote locations away from major centres of population. It is part of their appeal as resorts to which people have escaped from the pressures of everyday life and the pollution of cities. Britain's most northerly, westerly and easterly spas certainly conform to this pattern. Strathpeffer in the Scottish Highlands, Llandrindod Wells in mid-Wales and Woodhall Spa at the edge of the Lincolnshire Wolds stand in the middle of sparsely populated countryside, their huge hotels, grand villas and ornate public buildings seeming incongruous in their isolated rural settings. Many Continental

European spas are similarly tucked away. They are often literally at the end of the line when it come to access by rail, nowhere more so than the original Spa, which is reached by an ancient two-carriage train from Aachen that trundles through a wooded valley and makes its final halt at the terminus of Spa-Géronstère, named after one of the main sources and consisting of a single platform, a small shelter and a set of buffers.

The sources that provide spas with their *raison d'être* are also often hidden and secret. Water emerges mysteriously from the ground, having lain hidden for hundreds of thousands of years, forced up under pressure because of geological faults and rock fissures, sometimes in a trickle or a steady flow but often seething and steaming, gushing out in strong, pulsing ejaculations. Penetrating to these sources can be a profoundly mystical experience. I have felt this descending to the original spring at Baden bei Wien, discovered by the Romans and called the Römerquelle. It is reached by going through a door in a faceless modern municipal building behind the elegant Edwardian Summer Arena where operettas are performed. A steep flight of steps descends deep into the earth to arrive in a marble-tiled hall with a glass-covered dome under which the spring continually bubbles up as if from an enchanted cauldron. In many spas, it is difficult to find the source of the waters. They seep out of hidden fissures and swamps, concealed behind dense foliage or by a network of half-buried pipes and tanks which capture the precious water and channel it to bath houses and pump rooms.

The hiddenness of the sources of thermal waters has given rise to contrasting reflections. For some, it prompts thoughts of God, as in the inscription in the stained-glass window installed in 1888 in the hallway of the Royal Baths in Bath:

The spring from whence these waters flow
In the deep rock lies hid below,
So let thy bounty hidden be
And only God the giving see.

By contrast, early descriptions of spas often speak of their waters coming from 'the very bowels of the earth' and compare them to the infernal regions of the Underworld. There is often something rather Hell-like about their location and atmosphere. This was certainly the case with the original baths at Pfäfers near the modern Swiss spa of Bad Ragaz, which were located at the bottom of the precipitous Tamina Gorge. The thermal spring here, which emerges through rocks from an underground lake at a constant temperature of 36.5 degrees Celsius (98 degrees Fahrenheit) and a rate of seven million litres a day, making it Europe's most abundant thermal mineral water source, was supposedly first discovered around 1240 by birdcatchers hunting for ibis. Traversing the steep-sided cliffs where the birds nested, they noticed steam emerging from their base. Discounting the fear that they might encounter dragons in the murky depths below, they made the perilous descent to the bottom of the gorge where they found pools of hot water, which subsequent visitors found to be efficacious for relieving muscular pain and curing rheumatism and other conditions. For the first 300 years of their existence, the natural baths at Pfäfers could only be accessed via ropes with bathers being lowered several hundred feet down the sheer cliff face in baskets or slings (Plate 1). Even after a wooden staircase was built up the side of the gorge in 1543, the descent remained perilous and there were numerous accidents. Those brave enough to take a cure there are said to have remained for up to twelve days in the primitive baths hewn out of rock where, in the words of an observer in 1550, 'they sat in the dark like souls in St Patrick's Purgatory'. A visitor in 1630 described 'a horrible site of deepest solitude, similar to the Acheron or the Stygian swamps' (Croutier 1992: 144–5). Even today, when the source is accessed via a hair-raising four-kilometre bus journey down a twisting single-track road with a precipitous drop, followed by a 450-metre walk along a narrow pathway clinging to the side of the cliff wall with the Tamina river raging below, it remains a terrifying place with just a tiny chink of daylight far above relieving the gloom of the dark, dank, oppressive primeval atmosphere.

Other thermal water sources have been similarly compared to Hell over the years. In Richard Graves' 1773 comic romance, *The Spiritual Quixote*, a Bath landlord frightens one of his guests on his return from the baths by telling him that their heat 'was caused by a constant fire in the bowels of the earth, which had been burning ever since Noah's flood and would in time burn up the whole world' (Graves 1792: 350). An anonymous rhyme about Harrogate's highly sulphurous springs suggests demonic origins:

As Satan was flying over Harrogate's wells
His senses were charmed by the heat and the smells!
Said he, 'I don't know in what region I roam,
But I guess from the smell that I'm not far from home!'

Rather different evocations of Hell and the Underworld are conjured up in one of the key features of the cure at the Austrian spa of Bad Gastein where patients are taken on special trains deep into the nearby Böckstein mountain to lie for hours inhaling radon gas in tunnels originally dug by gold miners. The ancient mines were reopened during the Second World War by Hermann Goering to raise funds for the Nazi war effort and prisoners sent down to dig for gold reported their aches, pains and war wounds being mysteriously cured by the effects of the radioactive gas. The combination of the radioactivity, sweltering heat and humidity in the tunnels, known as the *Heilstollen*, is not to everyone's taste and there are a good many warnings about the feeling of suffocation and claustrophobia that may be experienced by those being taken into the bowels of the mountain to undergo this hidden and somewhat hellish cure.

Like the invisible radon gas used in the cure at Bad Gastein and at several other European spas, the chemical and mineral elements that play such an important role in the supposed therapeutic benefits of thermal waters are often hidden. Sometimes they are revealed by sight or smell – the reddish colour of the waters at Tunbridge Wells indicates that they are chalybeate, or iron-rich, while the strong whiff of rotten eggs that hangs around Harrogate points to the high sulphur content of the waters there. Unlike iron and sulphur, the third most common component found in thermal waters, sodium chlorine, which provides the saline sources found in many spas, is largely colourless and odourless, as are other minerals such as barium, magnesium and calcium. Only detailed chemical analysis reveals what is in the water.

Many of the therapeutic benefits associated with spa cures are also largely hidden. The water does its stuff out of sight, if not out of mind. This is especially the case with drinking-based cures where the emphasis is on cleansing, purging and washing out the system and effectively tackling digestive problems, constipation, diseased liver and urinary complaints. The after-effects of taking the waters cannot always be hidden, however. The strongly diuretic and laxative properties of the highly saline waters at Llandrindod Wells were reflected in the row of seventy-six toilets erected near the pump room. The therapeutic benefits of bathing in thermal waters are similarly hidden, being effected through the supposed penetration of mineral traces into the skin so that they reach the bloodstream and perform their healing work on vital organs, tissue and muscles. It is especially the unseen parts of the body which spas claim to treat – notably the intestines, sexual organs and nether regions. A patient taking a cure in Baden-Baden in the mid-nineteenth century described the doctor coming into his bedroom at five thirty in the morning and briskly announcing, '*Monsieur, nous allons visiter les entrails* [sic]' before proceeding 'to palp and palp the abdomen, looking grave and concentrated' and eventually exclaiming: '*Les entrails sont libres*' (Granville 2012: 81).

There are other hidden aspects of spa treatments. They are often carried out in private. Drinking the waters has always been, and remains, a largely communal activity, albeit one often undertaken in a rather hushed atmosphere of silent determination with little social interaction. Throughout the Middle Ages bathing was also communal and, following the example of the Romans, it was often the occasion for considerable conviviality and not a little sexual excitement. From the later eighteenth century onwards there was a growing tendency to take baths in private and the numerous spa treatments, including douches, massages, inhalations and increasingly complex therapies involving electrical and magnetic currents that proliferated in the nineteenth and twentieth centuries, were administered behind closed doors. Anyone visiting a spa for medical purposes today enters a secret world of long featureless corridors, off which are treatment rooms and cubicles hidden from public view. They generally have separate entrances from the more open and inviting recreational and 'wellness' areas of spa buildings. This is very clearly the case in the Gellért Baths in Budapest where those undergoing medical treatments are directed up a discreet and rather dingy set of side stairs by a sign saying 'Inhalatorium, Complex Physiotherapy and Curative Gymnastics'. They lead to a network of coldly clinical white-walled passages, reminiscent of hospital out-patient areas, filled with people sitting on plastic chairs, clutching their treatment plans and waiting for a therapist to usher them into his or her private demesne. The atmosphere could not be more different from the open, brightly coloured art deco halls of the main bath complex which is all that the many tourists and leisure bathers see.

There can also be a rather hidden aspect to the *Kurparks* which form the serious 'thermal zone' in several spas. It is not just that they tend to be sited off the main thoroughfares and away from the bustle of shopping streets and places of entertainment. They are often slightly gloomy spaces full of dark overhanging trees. In Bad Schwalbach in the Hesse region of Germany large signs at the entrance to the *Kurpark* bear the command '*Ruhe!*' (Quiet!). Looming over the north side are the high walls of one of the many clinics, which specialise in psychosomatic medicine as well as rehabilitation and the treatment of degenerative conditions. When

I walked through the park, I was conscious of pale, sad, shadowy faces peering down from tiny windows on the top floor of what looked all too like a prison. In Bad Ems, those undertaking prescribed medical cures are even more tucked away out of sight, being herded together in three huge and very ugly clinics surrounded by trees in the forbidding *Kurwald*, which is sited on the top of the cliffs above the town. It constitutes a hidden, self-contained abode of the sick far removed from the jolly world of weekend wellness packages in the hotels below (see page 259).

There is a more pervasive hidden side to spas which is a major theme of this book. It is well expressed in the German word *der Kurschatten*, literally the cure shadow, to which I was introduced by a German academic as we walked through the deserted streets of Bad Wildbad, a rather haunted spa town itself hidden away in the middle of the Black Forest. She told me that it signifies 'the shadow who is following you throughout your stay and disappears when you go home'. The word is generally used to describe the romantic and amorous dalliances that regularly took place in spas during their golden age, and perhaps much more occasionally still do today. Dictionary definitions range from the somewhat coy 'lady/gentleman friend met during a stay at a spa', through 'person at a health spa with whom one develops a relationship' and 'admirer at a health resort' to the rather more bold 'companion of the opposite sex picked up while on a cure'. The German Wikipedia entry on *der Kurschatten* states that 'it implies eroticism but the resulting relationship can also remain platonic'. Indeed, it can refer to a spa romance that never gets beyond the stage of imagination and fantasy. The phrase is expressed visually in a series of saucy German postcards showing older men chasing younger women and in the *Kurschattenbrunnen* sculptured in 1987 in the central square of the spa town of Bad Wildungen in North Hesse, Germany. A group of naked bathers are clustered close together in the centre of the fountain. In one of the pools around its base, an elderly naked man sits looking out towards a female figure walking past in a figure-hugging dress. Depending on the position of the sun, she casts a shadow over her admirer (Plate 11).

There were many reasons why those staying in spas seem to have been particularly susceptible to amorous dalliances and sexual encounters. The principle of romances on ocean liners, that 'what happens on board stays on board', pertained among those taking a cure, who were often without an accompanying spouse, spending anything from two or three weeks to several months away from home, and unlikely to meet their fellow *curistes* again. These circumstances were conducive to the formation of relationships and encouraged a belief that casual flings could be indulged in with no lasting consequences – although, as we shall see, several men and women came away from taking the waters with rather more than they had bargained for in the form of sexually transmitted diseases or pregnancies. Then there was the fact that bathing was often naked and mixed – one thing not hidden in spas was the human body. From Roman times until the present day, bath houses have been notorious as places for pick-ups and casual sexual encounters and in the Middle Ages many effectively functioned as brothels and became known as 'stew houses'.

Both male impotence and female sterility were prominent on the list of conditions which it was claimed were most successfully treated by a course of taking the waters internally and externally. Those suffering from the former complaint may perhaps sometimes have been stimulated into potency by the sight of the jets of thermal water that shot from the ground with huge force at several spas and which are difficult to describe without using language suggestive of male ejaculation. There is an unmistakable sexual as well as mystical note in this account by an English visitor to Karlsbad in the mid-nineteenth century of the *Sprudel* fountain which still excites visitors today:

The violent, lofty, constant and prodigal up-pourings of hot water out of the bowels of the earth, foaming in the midst of its clouds of vapour, rivetted me to the spot for some moments ...

What is it that imparts to this mysterious current that violent
impulse which makes it spring from the bosom of the earth,
with an upright jet, of eight or nine feet elevation and which
propels it, with convulsive and vehement throbs? ... In times
of darkness and superstition, man would have fallen prostrate
before, and adored, this unquiet and relentless agent which fills
the atmosphere with hot vapours and impetuously overruns
all the bounds by which art has vainly attempted to restrain its
endless throes. (Granville 2012: 102)

I have to say that the imagery of male ejaculation came to my mind
when I first saw the Coesa Spouter in Saratoga Springs State Park.
The water spurts intermittently from a piece of rubber tubing that
rides up and down in the middle of a lake looking from a distance
like a mini-Loch Ness Monster. An American lady viewing the same
spouter in the mid-nineteenth century was left with a rather different
impression. It inspired her to pen this improving ditty, which more
than makes up in high-minded moral sentiment for what it lacks in
poetic sophistication:

Oh water that doth mount on slender tip,
And spoutest up some thirty feet, through pole;
Oh Hope, learn thou a lesson from the water's lip,
Spout out, spout out, in peace from hollow soul.

This chaste female take on the thrusting vigour of spa waters
contrasts with the way that they were often marketed to women
desperate to conceive. As well as bathing in them, they were encouraged to play around a bit with the local men in case it was their
husbands who were the problem. A ballad published in 1678 described
the pleasures awaiting those who came to Tunbridge Wells:

Then you that hither childless come,
Leave your dull marriage behind you.

You'll never wish yourselves at home:
Our youth will be so kind to you.

The resident physician in Bad Ems in the mid-nineteenth century, Dr Celius, was well known for telling beautiful upper-class ladies that their illnesses would only be cured if they separated from their husbands. Among those who took his advice was Susan, Countess of Lincoln, who sparked off a major society scandal in 1848 by embarking on a disastrous affair there with Lord Walpole. There were plenty of other spa doctors who could be relied on to offer similar advice to those who felt themselves trapped in boring marriages.

The amatory possibilities inherent in spa cures have been a constant theme of writers. In 1592, the English traveller Fynes Moryson noted of those visiting Baden bei Zürich in Switzerland that 'many having no disease but that of love come hither for remedy, and many times find it' (Strachan 1962: 74). A treatise about the same spa published in 1739, which recounted the tale of an aristocrat who came with a broken leg and left with a nun whom he abducted, described the baths as 'a theatre of illicit pleasures' (Grenier 1985: 147). John Saxe's poem 'Pray, What Do They Do at the Springs' gave a candid sense of what went on in Saratoga Springs in the 1840s:

Now they stroll in the beautiful walks,
Or loll in the shade of the trees;
Where many a whisper is heard
That never is told by the breeze;
And hands are commingled with hands,
Regardless of conjugal rings;
And they flirt, and they flirt, and they flirt,
And that's what they do at the Springs!

Flirting in both North American and European spas often began as early as five or six in the morning when people gathered at the springs. Simply seeing women drink excited some men, like the one who was moved to verse as he watched a 'surpassingly beautiful lady' at the White Sulphur Springs in Virginia:

> She drinks – she drinks; behold the matchless dame;
> To her 'tis water – but to us 'tis flame

Another would-be poet employed more suggestive language as he envied 'the liquid she sips/Between her pulpy, swelling, ruby lips' (Chambers 2002: 137).

Several of those writing about spas suggested that they suited clandestine affairs and passionate couplings not just because of the sensuousness and steaminess of the waters but also because of the many beautiful walks and shady, secluded corners in their *Kurparks* which seemed almost to have been designed for illicit romance. In his description of Bad Homburg in the opening pages of his tale of spa seduction, 'Eugene Pickering', Henry James highlighted the *Kurpark*'s 'dusky woods' and the fact that even on a hot day 'you may walk about for a whole afternoon in unbroken shade' (James 1999: 36, 40). Ford Madox Ford, who himself knew a thing or two about spa romances, wrote in similar terms of Bad Nauheim's 'discreet shelters' (Ford 2008: 10).

Spas were favourite places for affairs and seductions both in real life and in fiction. They usually but not invariably involved older men and young women. The twenty-two-year-old courtesan, Marie Duplessis, later to be the model for Marguerite Gautier in Alexandre Dumas' *La Dame aux camélias* and Violetta in Verdi's *La traviata*, became the mistress of a wealthy seventy-year-old count while staying in Baden-Baden in the hope of curing her tuberculosis. Johann von Goethe regularly visited the spas of Bohemia to cure his gout, stomach problems and insatiable libido, pursuing numerous young women in Karlsbad and Marienbad including one who was his junior by more than fifty years (see pages 122 and 138). He dismissed his spa romances as mere *Äugelchen* (oglings) but the objects of his leering took a rather different view – one complained that 'he viewed the world as one big peep-show'.

German spas in particular became popular settings for seductions in nineteenth- and early twentieth-century novels. Among those who fell victim in Baden-Baden were the young bride seduced at the baths by an unscrupulous Italian marquis in Leo Tolstoy's *Family Happiness*, the innocent maiden beguiled into unhappy wedlock by a feckless lord in George Meredith's *The Amazing Marriage*, and the destitute lady's maid whisked off by the son of a prosperous American manufacturer in Theodore Dreiser's *Jennie Gerhardt*. Not all these fictional seductions involved older men having their wicked way with young women. The hero of Ivan Turgenev's *Smoke*, also set in Baden-Baden, was a naïve and recently engaged young farmer fatally attracted to and seduced by the older woman with whom he had been in love ten years earlier. Two novels set in Bad Homburg had a similar theme: Edmund Yates's *Black Sheep* chronicled the seduction of the married hero, Stewart Routh, by Mrs Ireton Bembridge, a predatory but beguiling New York socialite, while in Henry James's 'Eugene Pickering' the eponymous hero broke off his engagement and had a month-long affair with the widowed Madame Blumenthal who seduced him at the gaming table (see page 160). In Turgenev's novella *Spring Torrents* the naïve Sanin was seduced, and his engagement to his beloved scuppered, by the 'man-eating' Madame Polozova in Wiesbaden.

Several authors put their own experiences of *Kurschatten* into their novels. Ford Madox Ford based *The Good Soldier* on the adulterous affair on which he had embarked with fellow writer Violet Hunt in 1910. It began in Bad Nauheim and continued in Bad Homburg and Bad Schwalbach. The book is set in Bad Nauheim and painfully describes the adulterous relationship that develops between Florence Dowell and Edward Ashburnham, 'just exactly the sort of chap that you could have trusted your wife alone with' yet who shows himself 'a raging stallion forever neighing after his neighbour's womenkind' during the annual cures that they take with their respective spouses

(Ford 2008: 16). Stefan Zweig's short story 'The Burning Secret' (originally 'Brennendes Geheimnis'), which was turned into a silent film in 1923 and filmed again in 1933 and 1988, tells of a beautiful woman bringing her asthmatic adolescent son to the Austrian spa of Semmering for a cure. There they meet a suave, mysterious Austrian baron who first charms the boy with his stories and then seduces his mother. It was based on Zweig's own childhood experience in Marienbad where an older man befriended him only in order to get close to his mother. It has been suggested that Zweig's memories of this unhappy experience may have been the source of his deep-seated sexual inhibitions in adulthood.

Spas were favourite places for men to install their mistresses. Zulma Bouffar, the strikingly beautiful and flirtatious twenty-year-old singer with whom Jacques Offenbach was first infatuated when he saw her performing in the music hall in Bad Homburg, became his constant companion and lover during summers at Bad Ems, where he ran the music in the Marmorsaal concert hall, while his wife dutifully stayed at home in Paris with their children. It was not just men who entertained their lovers in spas while their spouses were at home. Eliza Potter, who ran a beauty salon in Saratoga Springs and wrote a book based on the confessions of her clients, described 'one beautiful and newly-married lady with an old rich husband' who pursued a lengthy affair during her stays there. Her husband would join her for weekends but when he departed on Monday morning to go back to work, 'her weekly consolation in the shape of a favourite lover' would arrive by train. Potter was intrigued by 'the sober dress and quiet habits of the lady when the poor old husband was by; and the transition to gaiety when the lover came'. She reported on another married woman who regularly threw dinner parties for 'her lover and a few female friends with their lovers' for which her husband footed the bill (Chambers 2002: 146).

Although the term der Kurschatten is usually taken to apply only to affairs and romances, it seems to me that it can be applied much more widely to the many other shadows so often cast over the lives and the minds of those staying in spas. As well as longing and lust, they included a heightening of the depression and melancholy already present in many of those seeking a cure, and an intense morbid introspection. One of the most visible and damaging *Kurschatten*, which features in many of the novels set in spas and exacted a terrible toll on those who succumbed to it, was addiction to the gambling provided in casinos and assembly rooms as the major diversion from the grim regime of the daily cure. No *Kurgast* perhaps succumbed more disastrously to the lure of the roulette wheel and the card tables, nor wrote about his addiction so powerfully, as Fyodor Dostoyevsky. His novel *The Gambler* (1867), set in the fictional German spa of Roulettenberg but based on his own experiences at Wiesbaden was, appropriately, tossed off in a little over a month to pay off some of the huge debts he had accumulated there and at Baden-Baden.

Other shadows fell across the elegant colonnades and grand hotels of Europe's watering places. Spas became places to which people escaped, or where they disappeared or were hidden away. Often this was to escape from unhappy marriages. Queen Marie Henriette of Belgium retreated to Spa in 1895 to get away from her husband, Leopold II, and his many mistresses – he subsequently at the age of sixty-five took up with a sixteen-year-old French prostitute. She spent the rest of her life there living in a house which became known as the Villa Royale, now the town museum. Although Napoleon Bonaparte himself was not a fan of any kind of bathing, famously writing to his wife Josephine, 'will be home in three weeks. Don't wash', four of the women most closely associated with him all sought refuge from failing marriages in the same French spa. His favourite sister Pauline, bored out of her mind by her husband, Prince Camillo Borghese, whom she had been forced to marry for diplomatic reasons, began a circuit of French *villes d'eaux* in 1807, taking in Plombières-les-Bains, Gréoux-les-Bains and Aix-les-Bains. She settled in Aix, bathing in donkey milk in a marble bath and cavorting with her new lover, Comte Auguste de Forbin. The street where she lived became known as the Rue des Soupirs, supposedly because of the sighs of her many suitors. The Empress Josephine took a cure at Aix in 1810 after Napoleon had divorced her for failing to produce an heir, despite having spent many weeks sitting in the hot springs at Plombières in an attempt to conceive. Her daughter Hortense also went to Aix after leaving her husband, Louis Bonaparte, King of Holland, to embark on a passionate affair with Charles de Flahaut. Napoleon's second wife, Marie-Louise, did not accompany him when he was exiled to Elba in 1815 but rather followed what was by now a family tradition and decamped to Aix where she began an affair with Count Adam von Neipperg.

The theme of escape from unhappy relationships is prominent in fictional accounts of spas. At the end of Anthony Trollope's novel *The Small House at Allington* Alexandrina Crosbie leaves her husband to make 'a long visit – a very long visit' to Baden-Baden (Trollope 1997: 564). It provides a socially acceptable form of separation, allowing them to remain married without having to see one another. In *Anna Karenina* Kitty Shcherbátsky is sent to a German spa to get over the emotional and physical breakdown caused by her rejection by Count Vronsky and her spurning of Konstantin Levin. Evelina Anville, the heroine of Fanny Burney's *Evelina*, takes herself off for a cure at the Bristol Hotwells, a spa in the Avon Gorge at Clifton, to recover after a terrible misunderstanding with Lord Orville, with whom she is still in love. Even before she has taken the waters, she finds herself much restored thanks to the beautiful prospect, the pure air and the 'weather very favourable to invalids'. However, the calm and serene atmosphere of the spa is broken when she is accosted and propositioned by three very rude and forward gentlemen on the way to the pump room. Throwing off her caddish pursuers, and placating the other female cure guests who are angry at her popularity, she is reunited with the gentle Lord Orville and they marry. In this account the spa has played an ambivalent role – healing and soothing, but also proving a hothouse of lust, passion and jealousy, while eventually letting virtue and

gentility prevail. Not all fictional accounts of escapes to spas involve
unhappy relationships. Jane and Elizabeth Purbeck's novel *Neville
Castle* describes an Italian marquis, about to be falsely accused of
treason, evading his persecutors by 'pretending to be attacked by an
indisposition for which his physician recommended a German spa'
(Purbeck 1802: 147).

Perhaps the most dramatic and well-publicised real-life use of a
spa as a hideaway occurred in 1926 when Agatha Christie fled to
Harrogate where she checked into a hotel in her husband's lover's
name and remained undetected for ten days while a nationwide
search tried to locate her (see page 222). The anonymity of spas
provided the perfect cover for several well-known figures to remain
incognito. Tsar Alexander II used the name Borodinski when he
stayed in Bad Ems, where he seems to have had his own *Kurschatten*
in the person of the enigmatic and beautiful Princess Katharina
Dolgoruki. Karl Marx checked in for a cure in Karlsbad under
the name 'Charles Marx, squire of London' in an attempt to avoid
the attentions of the police because his name had been linked to
riots in various European cities. For three years in the late 1880s
Queen Victoria spent three weeks in Aix-les-Bains in the summer
under the guise of the Countess of Balmoral and largely escaped
the prying attentions of journalists and others. While there she
acquired a French masseuse and a donkey, called Jacquot, whom
she brought back to pull her in a special wheelchair and also to
distribute Christmas presents to her grandchildren at Buckingham
Palace. Edward VII travelled to Marienbad as the Duke of Lancaster,
although his massive corporeal presence and pursuit of ladies around
the *Kurpark* made him recognisable everywhere as the English king.

Several of those who have been hidden away in spas have not gone
there of their own volition. The New Zealand author Katherine
Mansfield was packed off by her mother in 1909 to Bad Wörishofen
when she became pregnant out of wedlock and then walked out of
a hastily arranged marriage on the evening of the wedding because
of a lesbian affair. She turned her experiences there into a series

of short stories, *In a German Pension*, which give a vivid picture of the pettiness and ennui of life in a German *Kurort* (see page 208). Princess Alice of Battenberg, mother of Prince Philip, was diagnosed with schizophrenia following a mental breakdown in 1930 and shut up in sanatoria for six years, first in Kreuzlingen in Switzerland and then in the South Tyrolean spa of Merano, largely, it seems, because her husband, Prince Andrew of Greece, wanted her out of the way so that he could pursue his own amorous affairs in the south of France.

Stays in spas, whether for short or long periods, on a voluntary or an enforced basis, often induced a sense of boredom, lassitude and oppression. There are many accounts of the dull monotony of the carefully regulated and unchanging daily routine of drinking, promenading, bathing and resting. Alexis and Marie de Tocqueville, who visited Baden bei Zürich in 1836 in an effort to ease the latter's menstrual pains, declared themselves 'extremely bored' throughout their time there. Two years later, Grace Hunter noted in her diary during a six-week stay in Red Sulphur Springs, Virginia: 'Nothing could be more monotonous than the time spent here, and I fear as far as I am concerned unprofitable, both as respects mind and body, for besides feeling sick, and inert, I cannot feel as if I was settled or give myself up to any useful employment. I am too stupid, so dull, and often so sleepy, I hardly know what to think of myself' (Hunter 1838). Washington Irving summed up his stays at various American springs as 'a life of alternate lassitude and fatigue, of laborious dissipation and listless idleness, of sleepless nights and days spent in that dozing insensibility which ever succeeds them'. He worried that their growing popularity among the commercial and professional classes was contributing to a culture of idleness and sapping America's moral fibre and entrepreneurial drive (Chambers 2002: 115). On the whole, British spa-goers were less inclined to such moralistic observations but they were equally gripped by a pervasive sense of ennui and tedium. Oscar Wilde wrote (in French) to a friend from Bad Homburg in 1892, 'I am enormously bored here.' The previous year, Arthur Sullivan had summed up his first spa cure, taken over thirty days in Contrexéville in an attempt to ameliorate his recurrent kidney problems, in similar terms:

> There is a constant delirious whirl of dullness here, the counterpart of which is only to be found in England at a Young Men's Christian Association weekly evening recreation. I am up at 6am, *masse'd* and douched, and drink 6 pints of the mineral water, walking all the time until breakfast at 10. Nothing more to eat and drink till 6 when we dine – then to bed at 10, to resume the same existence at 6 next morning. I need scarcely tell you that the two meals are the two great events of the day. (Bradley 2010: 19)

This particular spa shadow has also been well caught by novelists. The first description of the *curistes* in Guy de Maupassant's *Mont-Oriol*, set in an imaginary newly constructed *ville d'eau* called Enval in the Auvergne and based on the author's own experience of taking a cure at Châtel-Guyon, portrays them slowly pacing up and down drinking water or sitting idly on benches in the casino grounds and notes that 'their minds seemed a blank, and they themselves paralysed, bored to extinction, by the deadly monotony that characterizes all health resorts' (Maupassant: 20). In *The Good Soldier*, the narrator, John Dowell, initially describes the life of himself and his fellow *Kurgäste* at Bad Nauheim as 'a minuet', so-called because 'we knew where to go, where to sit, which table we unanimously should choose; and we could rise and go … without a signal … always to the music of the Kur orchestra.' He later comes to realise that 'it wasn't a minuet that we stepped; it was a prison – a prison full of screaming hysterics' (Ford 2008: 11). Something of the same sense of entrapment is captured and conveyed in a very different though no less emphatic way in the later operettas of Franz Lehár, penned as he sat in the dark oppressive study on the top floor of his villa on the banks of the River Traun in Bad Ischl. It is perhaps nowhere more powerfully expressed than in *Der Zarewitsch*, with its libretto by two writers who also lived in the Austrian spa town. Gloriously romantic and escapist, it is also full of wistful longing, melancholy and a sense of impermanence and mortality. The tortured heir to the Russian throne, a character written like all Lehár's late romantic tenor roles for Richard Tauber, who lived in a nearby villa just along the Traun, feels imprisoned in a gilded cage as he sings of his intense loneliness: '*Allein, wieder allein*' (alone, again alone). Like so many of Lehár's songs, and indeed so much of the music played in *Kurkonzerte*, it has a wistful, bitter-sweet quality of yearning and longing, hinting at repressed and unreconciled feelings.

The loneliness often felt by those taking a spa cure was part of a more pervasive sense of melancholy that cast another long and lingering *Kurschatten*. Many came seeking relief for what would now be described as depression but for a long time was called melancholia, or sometimes referred to as nervous neuralgia or an attack of the vapours. In a lingering hangover from the ancient idea that disease is caused by an imbalance of humours in the body or bloodstream, the condition was famously defined in Robert Burton's *Anatomy of Melancholy*, first published in 1621, as one 'which goes and comes upon every small occasion of sorrow, need, sickness, trouble, fear, grief, passion, or perturbation of the mind, any manner of care, discontent, or thought, which causes anguish, dullness, heaviness and vexation of spirit' (Burton 1847: 93). While no one was immune from what was an inevitable aspect of mortality, melancholia became serious when it took on the character of 'a habit, a chronic disease and a settled humour' which could verge on insanity (Burton 1847: 94). Burton, who singled out two specific conditions in his influential study – lovers' melancholy and religious melancholy – did not specifically recommend spa treatments for melancholics, preferring rather to focus on exercise, diet, purging, bloodletting and various potions. Later medical treatises, however, did advocate them as an effective cure for melancholia and many spas put it high in the list of ailments for the treatment of which their waters were particularly effective.

Melancholia continued to be recognised as a distinct medical condition well into the nineteenth century and many doctors sent patients who were deemed to be suffering from it for spa cures. Unfortunately, these often made their depression worse. Indeed, melancholy came to be recognised as a specific condition that took hold of those taking a cure. The French novelist Octave Mirbeau, who took a cure in Luchon in 1897, identified it as '*la mélancolie des villes d'eaux*' and noted that it made *curistes* 'like poor blind beasts spin round and round on the merry-go-round of their boredom' (Mirbeau 1977: 79). A sad testament to this were the attempted suicides that took place in spas. *The History of Tom Jones*, which Henry Fielding wrote on the basis of his own experiences of living in Bath in the 1740s, includes a harrowing account of the rescue by the eponymous hero of a fellow cure guest who jumped into the water in an effort to end his miserable life. In 1826, when Karl van Beethoven, nephew of the composer, decided to take his life it was to Baden bei Wien that he went, taking with him a pair of pistols and gunpowder. He walked through the Helenental valley, climbed to the ruins of Rauhenstein, where he had often gone with his uncle, and put both pistols to his temple. The first bullet flew harmlessly past while the second ripped through his flesh but did not damage his skull. He was later found lying in the ruins, badly wounded but alive.

Those who fled to spas to get away from unhappy situations or escape from their demons could find themselves even more trapped and desperate in their oppressive atmosphere. Helen Gladstone, sister of the Liberal prime minister, first embarked on what would prove to be a disastrous round of German *Kurorte* when she took a long cure in Bad Ems in 1838 to try to escape the constricting confines of her home in Scotland where she lived alone with her father. She followed this with a visit to Baden-Baden where she fell in love with and became engaged to a Russian-Polish count whose parents subsequently forbade the marriage, plunging her into deep depression. While taking an extended cure at Baden-Baden in 1845, she became addicted to opium. Her brother went out with the hope of bringing her home but found she was almost beyond help. On one occasion, after taking 300 drops of laudanum and becoming partially paralysed, she had to be held down by force while leeches were applied. Another time he discovered that she had drunk the best part of a bottle of eau de cologne mixed with water. She often locked the door of her room for days on end, hiding herself away in misery and shame. As he lived through eight gloomy weeks witnessing such scenes and watching his sister spiralling downwards, Gladstone found that both the family situation and the whole atmosphere of the fashionable *Kurort* induced in him a morbid introspection. Overwhelming feelings of guilt, especially in matters sexual, led him to intense self-examination and he drew up a memorandum of his own depravity, listing the channels through which sexual temptation came to him, the times when he was especially receptive, the chief actual dangers and the remedies. His main sin seems to have been reading pornography. Here, in what his biographer Roy Jenkins called 'this budget of guilt' (Jenkins 1995: 101), was a *Kurschatten* of a particularly obsessive and intense kind. Interestingly, the ambience and the waters of another well-known spa had a very different effect on Gladstone's great rival, Benjamin Disraeli. He wrote to Lady Londonderry in 1856 while on one of his many visits to Spa: 'I was so lethargically disposed the whole year that many things escaped my wearied life. The suppressed gout, at which you laughed, at length brought me here where, after a few weeks, I have found renovation in its bright fountains, and brown baths of iron waters' (Aldous 2007: 99).

Perhaps the difference between the two men's experiences is partly explained by the fact that Disraeli was taking a cure, which was apparently successful, while Gladstone was simply waiting around while his sister abused herself with drugs. The experience of taking a cure was bad enough in terms of its unpleasantness and excruciating boredom but being stuck in a spa for weeks while a family member or friend was taking one was even worse. In *The Good Soldier*, John Dowell graphically describes how he feels being marooned in Bad Nauheim through the hot summer of 1904 while his wife, Florence, is undergoing a cure:

> I don't know how it feels to be a patient at one of these places. I never was a patient anywhere. I daresay the patients get a home feeling and some sort of anchorage in the spot. They seem to like the bath attendants, with their cheerful faces, their air of authority, their white linen. But for myself, to be at Nauheim gave me a sense – what shall I say? – a sense almost of nakedness – the nakedness that one feels on the sea-shore or in any great open space. I had no attachments, no accumulations.
>
> I could find my way blindfolded to the hot rooms, to the douche rooms, to the fountain in the centre of the quadrangle where the rusty water gushes out. I know the exact distances. And now you understand that, having nothing in the world to do – but nothing whatever! I fell into the habit of counting my footsteps. (Ford 2008: 27–8)

Spas are places of stark contrasts and apparent contradictions, at once heavens and hells. They come closer than most other human settlements to being planned Utopias, created for healing, well-being and the pursuit of pleasure. Trading in dreams and fantasies of eternal youth, with their extravagant fairy-tale rococo and baroque architecture, and their host of diversions and entertainments, they are the true precursors and prototypes of Disney World and today's theme parks. Yet they can also be hellish. Added to the shadows of depression, loneliness and introspection is the physical unpleasantness of joining sweaty, smelly fellow bathers in steamy, sulphurous baths, an experience which put visitors to both Vichy and Bath in mind of Purgatory (see pages 27 and 76). The high-pressure douches spraying hot sulphurous water on *curistes* at

Aix-les-Bains were known as 'the showers of Hell' and the bathing establishment there even called the section with individual bathing cabins '*la division d'enfer*'.

The experience of bathing in thermal waters could be heavenly in one spa and hellish in another. This contrast is well brought out in the writings of the somewhat eccentric Italian-born and London-based physician Augustus Granville, who felt a mission to convince the sceptical British of the benefits of Continental balneotherapy and spa medicine and looked forward to the time when 'mineral waters will take the place of the perpetual drugging so injuriously prevalent in London' (Granville 2012: 150). The journals that he wrote during his extensive tours of the German *Kurorte* in the mid-1830s give one of the most vivid impressions of European spas in their golden age and will be much quoted in this book. Here he is in mystical vein describing the sensuous and spiritual delights of a bath he took in Wildbad:

> This soothing effect of the water, as it came over me, up to the throat, transparent like the brightest gem or aquamarine, soft, genially warm, and gently murmuring, I shall never forget. Millions of bubbles of gas rose from the sand and played around me, quivering through the lucid water as they ascended, and bursting at the surface. The sensation produced by these, with their tremulous motion, like the much vaunted effect of titillation in animal magnetism, is not to be described. It partakes at once of tranquility and exhilaration; of the ecstatic state of a devotee, blended with the repose of an opium eater. The head is calm, the heart is calm, every sense is calm; yet there is neither drowsiness, stupefaction nor numbness; for every feeling is freshened, and the memory of worldly pleasures keen and sharp. But the operations of the moral as well as the physical man are under the spell of some powerfully tranquilising agent. It is the human tempest, lulled into all the delicious playings of the ocean's afterwaves. (Granville 2012: 43)

On the same 1836 trip, a visit to the communal baths at Teplitz in Bohemia, where the water temperature was 45 degrees Celsius (113 degrees Fahrenheit) and the steam made it difficult to see very much, left Granville with a very different impression:

> I could perceive that both the men and women who were bathing had been recently cupped, or had had leeches applied to their backs, their shoulders, or their chests, and that blood was streaming from the wounds, fresh and free, into the water. These poor creatures cannot enter the water, on account of its great heat, without first losing blood, or they would expose themselves to serious accidents. Some were lying down in the water; others standing up; a few were playing and gamboling about; while many were engaged in rubbing one another. The greater number of the men and women were stripped of all clothes; but a few wore a small handkerchief round their waists. The whole spectacle reminded me strongly of those fiery pictures of Purgatory which one meets at the door of almost every church in Italy. (Granville 2012: 141)

This contrast is reflected in the quality and character of the waters themselves. They can be sweet, crystal clear, flowing swiftly and giving every appearance of a life-giving tonic and elixir. They can equally be dirty, brackish, evil-smelling, spitting out of rusty pipes choked by a build-up of mineral deposits or the vegeto-animal matter which leaves an eerie green-coloured sediment in the bottoms of baths and drinking glasses and is evocatively described in German as *Badeschleim*. It is often the most unpleasant-looking and evil-smelling water, discoloured and full of gunky slime, that is the most effective in bathing and drinking treatments. It is all too easy to be put off drinking or bathing in thermal mineral waters by their appearance or smell. The fact is that, in the reassuring words of a notice positioned above the Kneipp foot baths in the spa of the Nové Lázně hotel in Mariánské Lázně, as Marienbad is now called, 'Dank deposits from the minerals advance effect of the therapeutics.'

I was first made aware of this on a visit to Ilidža just a few miles from Sarajevo in what is now Bosnia but was then Yugolsavia, in the early 1980s. Walking a few hundred yards from the modern Hotel Terme, following the smell of rotten eggs and what sounded like cackling geese or intermittent Morse code, I came to a circular concrete tub into which rusty pipes were discharging pulsating bursts of steaming, sulphurous water. The scene struck me as a stage designer's vision of Hell. The tub was discoloured and filled with greenish slime and the ground around was swampy and oozing with steaming bubbles and springs. On one side, half hidden by dank undergrowth, the old bath house, a long low ochre-coloured building, stood derelict. On the other, a network of rusting pipes and valves housed in cracked concrete ducts carried the sulphurous water to the hotel and a drab clinic where it was bathed in by those suffering from rheumatism and sterility. A steady stream of local people were making their way through the dank undergrowth to the tub, cupping their hands in the evil-smelling slime and washing their faces. Undeterred by the rotting corpse of a fox in the bowl of the tub, several drank a mouthful of the water and others filled up bottles from the rusty pipe. They looked for all the world like medieval pilgrims venerating a sacred if distinctly unprepossessing shrine. It was clear that what for me seemed like the water of death was for them the water of life.

Spas are, indeed, simultaneously places of life and death, of vitality and decay and of well-being and sickness. The thrusting, pulsating geysers and the warm saline waters promise sexual potency and fecundity, an end to barrenness and sterility. The accent is on cure and improvement – nowadays on the ubiquitous 'wellness' – yet the wrinkled bodies sitting in the baths demonstrate all too eloquently that the Second Law of Thermodynamics cannot be gainsaid or reversed. Despite all their glitz and glamour, spas are in many ways depressing places; by their very nature and purpose, they are resorts of the sick and the dying. The nineteenth-century Irish writer Charles Lever, who noted 'the depressing influence which

streets full of pale faces suggest' and 'the melancholy derivable from
a whole promenade of cripples', was right in his verdict that 'there
is something indescribably sad in these rendezvous of ailing people
from all parts of Europe' (Lever 1894: 356). Spas have always
disproportionately attracted the infirm and the elderly – Turgenev
described Wiesbaden as home to 'a heavy concentration of retired
people' – and are even more so now when they are full of clinics
and nursing homes packed with wheelchairs and Zimmer frames.
They have long been places where people go to die. It is fitting that
Nikolai Gogol went to Marienbad in 1839 in search of inspiration
for his novel *Dead Souls* and that in nearby Karlsbad (now Karlovy
Vary) one of the most prominent leaflets in the tourist information
office is a guide to the town cemetery and its personalities.

There are other striking contrasts in the make-up of spas. They are
places which combine spirituality and sensuality, at once enchanted
and demonic. Guy de Maupassant described them in *Mont-Oriol* as
'the only true fairylands left upon the earth – you would really think
that the springs were not so much mineralized as bewitched'. He
also wrote of their commercial exploitation and the unscrupulous
ways in which they promote their supposed cures. Several spas
had religious origins in holy wells and long retained a mystical
and spiritual quality. Others became known principally for their
carnal and sybaritic pleasures. There is also a contrast between their
outward respectability and the gossip and scandals that bubble below
the surface just as steamily as the underground thermal waters. Spas
became a byword for propriety and slightly disapproving bourgeois
morality, with 'Disgusted of Tunbridge Wells' penning letters to
the *Daily Telegraph* from the Regency villas on Mount Ephraim and
Mount Sion, retired colonels in Cheltenham huffing and puffing
about the state of the nation, and fur-clad matrons tut-tutting on the
subject of declining moral standards while partaking of cream cakes
in the Café Zauner in Bad Ischl or walking their Pekinese dogs along
the Lichtentaler Allee in Baden-Baden. At the same time the casinos
and grand hotels of the most fashionable *Kurorte* and *villes d'eaux*

offered a glitzy menu of gambling, gourmandising, girls, gaiety and gossip until the early hours.

To some extent this combination made spas dens of hypocrisy. This is certainly how they tended to be portrayed in novels, especially from the mid-nineteenth century onwards. Those writing about them often also alluded to their falseness and artificiality, with everything being too perfect and having the feeling of being manicured rather than natural. Gérard de Nerval, the French writer and poet who spent much time in Baden-Baden, described its long avenue of poplars as being like a theatre curtain revealing 'a scene arranged as for a pastoral opera' and commented that 'one is struck first and foremost by the impression that the whole landscape has an artificial air. The trees are trimmed, the houses are painted, the mountains are vast canvases hanging on stretchers' (de Nerval 1928: 52). In *The Good Soldier*, John Dowell complained that in Bad Nauheim 'one is too polished up' and described how 'Whilst poor Florence was taking her morning bath, I stood upon the carefully swept steps of the *Englischer Hof*, looking at the carefully arranged trees in tubs upon the carefully arranged gravel whilst carefully arranged people walked past in carefully calculated gaiety, at the carefully calculated hour' (Ford 2008: 27). Everything was too pretty, too tame and too predictable. Lady Wolseley, wife of the most famous and most swashbuckling soldier in late Victorian Britain, made a similar observation about Marienbad in a letter to a friend: 'This place would bore you to death. It is extremely pretty, just like the scenery of an operetta, but the performers are those of a burlesque, grotesque from fat' (Bradley 2010: 29).

Lady Wolseley was not the only person to make the comparison with operetta. In 1867 Edmond and Jules de Goncourt described the chalets erected in Vichy by Napoleon III (supposedly to house his mistresses) as looking as though they belonged to a comic opera, while in his 1975 novel, *Villa Triste*, which is partly set in a mythical *ville d'eau* based on Évian, Patrick Modiano identifies the charm of such places as deriving from their operetta-like décor. In my book *Water Music*, I suggest that operetta, classically defined by Franz Lehár as 'something to be diverted by and then forgotten', is the quintessential musical expression of spa life and culture (Bradley 2010: 28). It is not surprising that so many operetta composers found spas congenial and fruitful places to work. Nor is it a coincidence that the two most popular operettas of all time, *Die Fledermaus* and *Die Lustige Witwe* (*The Merry Widow*) should have been respectively set and composed in a spa. *Die Fledermaus* was set in 'a spa near Vienna', almost certainly Baden bei Wien, where the librettist, Richard Genée, was based when he wrote it in 1874. Johann Strauss wrote much of the music while staying in his villa in the neighbouring spa of Bad Vöslau. Lehár wrote the score of *Die Lustige Witwe* during stays in Bad Ischl, which was also the home of its librettist, Victor Léon, and became the centre for European operetta composition in the first three decades of the twentieth century (see page 211).

Like operettas, spas were often accused of dealing in light trivialities, promoting an appealing but ultimately shallow feel-good factor and encouraging casual flirting and short-lived affairs rather than deep and lasting relationships. Writing in 1843, the American journalist Francis Grund saw one of their great advantages as being 'that you may eat, drink, play, talk and dance with a person at a watering-place, without being obliged ever to recognize the person again', a view echoed thirty-four years later in an article in *Chambers' Journal*: 'At such places as Ems and the various bathing-springs abroad, acquaintances are easily formed. Even if they are not always unexceptionable, they serve to pass the time, and when you leave, you are not likely ever to meet your friends of the summer again' (Morgan 2014: 294, 299).

Even if it was only at a superficial level and on a transient basis, spas throughout their golden age allowed social interaction between people from a wide variety of backgrounds and nationalities and with differing motivations for being there. 'Such a diversified gallery of portraits I have never seen grouped together,' a visitor to Saratoga

Springs in the mid-1850s observed, 'invalids in search of health, maidens in search of husbands, widows disconsolate, young men inclined to matrimony, politicians looking for votes' (Chambers 2002: 80–1). The fact that everyone was after something perhaps helps to explain another characteristic of spas: that they often seem to bring out the worst in people and encourage selfishness and a lack of concern for others. Those who came as invalids desperate for a cure tended already to be self-absorbed and gripped by what Charles Lever identified as 'the egotism of sickness'. Far from fostering a community of suffering, the company of so many ill people tended to lead either to jealousy about the progress of others or self-satisfaction about one's own state compared to the rest. Those, increasingly the majority, who came to spas in a relatively healthy state were equally if not more narcissistic, being almost wholly focused on pleasure-seeking among the many entertainments and diversions on offer. They shunned the sick, whom they saw as an embarrassing blot on an otherwise perfect landscape, and were in return eyed with envy by those who were genuinely ill. In my experience, it remains the case today that very few acts of altruism are carried out in spas. There is nothing comparable to the gentle priority given to the sick at Lourdes, a very different kind of healing place also based on water. Rather the whole atmosphere encourages everyone, whether desperate or decadent, to focus on and think about themselves.

Several writers who stayed in spas described their shame at being in such places. This was a constant theme of Dostoyevsky's letters from the German *Kurorte* where he gambled away his own and other people's money. Confessing his addiction to Baden-Baden's pleasures despite regarding it 'as a hovel and a place of ill-repute', Gérard de Nerval added, 'I am ashamed that God should see me here.' The German spas played a rather shameful role in the build-up to the Second World War, with Jewish *Kurgäste* being stigmatised and excluded, eugenics experiments being carried out in the bath houses and SS officers sleeping with specially-picked blonde women in the *Kurhotels* to propagate a 'pure' Aryan race. In the war itself, the Queen of the French *villes d'eaux* was chosen as the headquarters of Marshal Pétain's collaborationist government, giving the name Vichy an aura of stigma and shame that lasts to this day. Chosen partly because of its large number of grand hotels and thermal establishments, which could be used for government offices, it reinforced the image of spas as not very nice places.

Yet perhaps in their very shadiness and shame spas provide one of the truest reflections of the human condition, stripping naked souls as well as bodies. As Jery Melford reflected about Bath in Tobias Smollett's *The Expedition of Humphry Clinker*: 'Here a man has daily opportunities of seeing the most remarkable characters of the community. He sees them in their natural attitudes and true colours; descended from their pedestals, and divested of their former draperies, undisguised by art and affectation' (Smollett 1990: 47). There is nothing like sitting naked and steaming in a communal bath tub for washing away pride and pretension.

The biggest contrast and tension to be found in spas, which will be a major theme throughout this book, is that between health and hedonism. It was a constant theme of those who wrote about them during their long golden age. For the mid-nineteenth-century Russian writer, Mikhail Saltykov-Shchedrin, 'the official attraction of these resorts lies in the curative strength of their mineral springs and the restorative properties of the surrounding mountain air. The unofficial attraction is the endless revelry implied by a mass influx of idle and highly solvent people' (Morgan 2014: 88). Charles Lever had a characteristically witty Irish take on the juxtaposition of these two seemingly incompatible attractions which spas provided, and the very different kind of clientele drawn by each of them:

It was a strange ordinance of the age that made watering-places equally the resort of the sick and the fashionable, the dyspeptic and the dissipated. One cannot readily see by what magic chalybeates can minister to a mind diseased, nor how sub-carbonates and proto-chlorides may compensate to the faded spirit of an *ennuyée* fine lady for the bygone delights of the London or Paris season; much less, through what magnetic influence gambling and gossip can possibly alleviate affections of the liver, or roulette be made a medical agent in the treatment of chronic rheumatism. (Lever 1894: 355)

The fact was that spas were principally resorted to by two distinct groups of people who had widely different motivations and expectations. William Cobbett distinguished them when he described the clientele in Cheltenham in 1821 as consisting of 'the lame and the lazy, the gormandizing and guzzling, the bilious and the nervous'. Spas attracted equally the desperate and the decadent but there was generally little intermingling between them. Granville found plenty of the former on his 1836 tour round the spas of Germany and Austria. He met a young man from Hamburg who had lost the use of his right arm and leg and who had tried every kind of bath in numerous different *Kurorte*, including plunging into a tub filled with the skins and entrails of recently slaughtered animals, but all in vain until he took thirty-five baths in Bad Gastein and was restored to full health. At Bad Gastein he also encountered a sixty-five-year-old priest taking his twentieth bath of the morning in a desperate effort to cure himself of being unable to walk. But there were also rather more *Kurgäste* who were bent simply on pleasure and had no real interest in the medical aspects of their cures. This, he found, was especially true of Baden-Baden, which he felt could best be described as 'a medical as well as a fashionable spa', and where there were 'many thousand idlers, who devote just one hour, in every four-and-twenty, to the one great object, health; and two-thirds of the remaining time to pleasure and dissipation. These, more than the operations of bathing and drinking the mineral water, are the motives of the majority of those who visit Baden' (Granville 2012: 30).

These two worlds, of health and hedonism, desperation and decadence, existed in parallel with little if any overlap between them.

The Russian novelist Mikhail Lermontov described the clientele at a fashionable Caucasian spa in 1840 as being made up of two distinct groups, both of whom left much to be desired: 'Those who drink the waters in the morning are inert – like all invalids, and those who drink the wines in the evening are unendurable – like all healthy people!' (Lermontov 1912: 174). In similar vein, Yates's *Black Sheep* featured the contrasting figures of Harriet Routh, the faithful and dutiful English wife who, although she disliked Bad Homburg intensely, dutifully committed herself to a regular water-drinking regime, and Mrs Bembridge, the brash American seductress, who was never seen anywhere near the waters but rather frequented the casino and the shady paths in the *Kurpark*. It was by providing the facilities for these contrasting lives to be led in parallel and largely independent of each other that spas solved the conundrum posed by Charles Lever when he asked, 'How can the same tone of society please the mirthful and the melancholy?' (Lever 1894: 356).

Another contrast that struck several visitors to spas was that between the health of the attendants at the baths and springs and the pitiable condition of the invalids who frequented them. It made a strong impression on Tolstoy while he was in Baden-Baden, and he put it into a passage in *Anna Karenina* when Prince Shcherbátsky visits his daughter Kitty while she is taking a cure in Bad Soden: 'The nearer one came to the Spring the more often one met sick people, whose appearance seemed yet sadder amid the customary well-ordered conditions of German life.' Kitty had been so long in the spa that she 'was no longer struck by this contrast' but for her father, 'the radiance of the June morning, the sounds of the band playing a fashionable and merry valse, and particularly the appearance of the sturdy maid-servants, seemed improper and monstrous in contrast with all those melancholy living corpses collected from all parts of Europe.' It made him feel 'awkward and ashamed of his powerful stride and his large healthy limbs'. Indeed, 'he almost had the feeling that might be caused by appearing in company without clothes' (back to the theme of nakedness again) and, even though its waters had cured his daughter from tubercular disease, his overwhelming impression of the spa was of 'a very sad place' (Tolstoy 1958: 257–8).

Although they largely existed in separate parallel worlds, health and hedonism were brought together in close proximity in the physical layout of many spas. The casino was sited next to the bath house and the assembly rooms with their dance floors next to the pump room with its drinking fountains. In the thermal establishment at Enval as described in *Mont-Oriol*, 'medical waters, douches and baths were available on one storey; beer, liqueurs and music on the other' (Maupassant: 9). Originally, the diversions and entertainment were provided for those who were genuinely focused on health and taking the cure in an attempt to mitigate some of the excruciating boredom and physical unpleasantness that it entailed. There was only so much punishment by water that *curistes* could stand and distractions were devised to take their mind off their illness and the often rather brutal treatments that were prescribed for them. Among the first to be introduced were the bands of musicians who played early in the morning around the drinking fountains. Then there were the cafés and shops selling cream cakes, pastries, ice creams and other highly calorific delights designed to take away the bitter after-taste of the evil-smelling water. Such was the origin of famous *Konditorei* like Zauners in Bad Ischl and Café König in Baden-Baden. In 1840, John Farrah invented and started selling a particularly sweet toffee, similar to both butterscotch and barley sugar, to clear the palate of the putrid taste of Harrogate's sulphurous water. Original Harrogate Toffee is still made in a factory in the town and sold at Farrah's Olde Sweet Shop at the bottom of Montpellier Parade near the old royal baths. Spa wafers with the consistency of ice-cream cones, known as *oplatky* in Czech and *Oblaten* in German and still sold in Karlovy Vary and Mariánské Lázně, have a similar origin, having been first developed in the 1850s for *Kurgäste* to munch on as they took their morning and early-evening promenades with their special drinking cups around the fountain colonnades. These little hedonistic touches made the cure at least a bit more bearable. For some spa-goers the sweetmeats seem to have been the main attraction. The Aga Khan is said to have spent the season at Baden-Baden largely so that he could guzzle the ninety-eight varieties of patisserie available there.

Increasingly as spas prospered and developed, those coming to them purely for pleasure outnumbered those who were genuinely taking a cure. As early as 1674 a character in a comedy about an imaginary French *ville d'eau* reflected: 'One plays, one dances, one laughs, that's what it is to take the waters. For every four who drink, there are usually twenty others who have come only in search of amusement' (Grenier 1985: 151). Washington Irving noted in 1807 that whereas visiting the Springs of North America 'originally meant nothing more than relief from pain and sickness', they had now become 'careless places of resort where invalidism mattered little' (Chambers 2002: 75). As the nineteenth century progressed, the balance swung more and more in favour of hedonism over health, although the latter remained a convenient and respectable cover for baser motives. In an article entitled 'An Evening in a Caucasian Spa in 1824', Alexander Bestuzhev-Marlinskii asked: 'Why are we all here? Everyone will say: to take a cure. But aside from this many have incidental or even primary aims. Some come to dissipate themselves in love affairs; some to make themselves respectable through marriage; others to redeem the injustices of fortune at the card table' (Morgan 2014: 42). A fellow Russian journalist, Nikolai Grech, wrote from Baden-Baden, in 1835: 'The mineral waters are the last thing people think about. No one talks about illnesses. They come here to enjoy themselves, to play roulette, to socialise with their friends' (Morgan 2014: 80). In the same year the English eccentric William Beckford found Bad Ems to be 'full of idlers and billiard players' and Augustus Granville reported from Baden-Baden, 'That there are invalids among the many thousands who flock yearly to this spa, is undeniable. That the larger number of those who go thither have other objects than the pursuit of health, is equally certain' (Granville 2012: 26). Visiting the same *Kurort* in 1843, Gogol noted 'there is no one here who is seriously ill – they all come to enjoy themselves.'

There was a third important category of spa guest who was neither seriously ill nor simply bent on pleasure. Gogol himself belonged to it, coming to Baden-Baden preoccupied by the state of his bowels but without any significant ailment. He was a classic hypochondriac – and it is that condition which, alongside health and hedonism, forms the third major theme of this book. Hypochondria started out as a recognised physical condition. The word derives from *hypochondrium*, an anatomical term for the upper part of the abdomen containing the liver, gall bladder and spleen. Until well on in the eighteenth century hypochondria was seen as an ailment caused by imbalances in the stomach and digestive system. It came to be widely considered as nervous in origin, and so to some extent a disease of the mind, and was associated with symptoms ranging from too much spit to rumbling in the guts. It was closely related to melancholia, with both being regarded as a consequence of imbalance of bodily humours. The *hypochondrium* was seen as the seat of melancholy and source of the vapours that caused morbid feelings.

Patients diagnosed with hypochondria were often prescribed spa cures by their doctors. When in 1793 Erasmus Darwin, a physician who was regarded as something of an expert on the condition, identified twenty-two-year-old Tom Wedgwood as suffering from what he called hypochondriasis, he recommended the brilliant scientist, who was a member of the famous pottery family, to take the Harrogate waters. Tom's condition did not improve and in 1802 he was referred to another leading doctor, Matthew Baillie, who made a similar diagnosis on the basis of symptoms which provide a classic definition of hypochondria: 'He has a disrelish for the common amusements of society, and takes little interest in those pursuits which formerly used to engage his mind. His attention is almost entirely absorbed in watching his health, and minutely scrutinising every feeling of the body. The bowels are very torpid, the food he takes does not nourish the body, and he has in some measure lost the usual propensity towards the other sex' (Burman: 52). Baillie went on to note that 'hypochondriasis is very apt to last long and is but very little under the influence of medicine' and to suggest that Tom 'should endeavour as much as he can to amuse his mind among objects which are new and interesting and by travelling in foreign countries' (Burman: 53).

It was precisely such diversion, novelty and opportunity for travel that spas provided and it was not surprising that they appealed so much to hypochondriacs and made a speciality of treating them. Tunbridge Wells advertised its waters as being especially efficacious for those suffering from 'hypochondriacal and hysterical fits'. Alongside the many spa-goers with rheumatism and arthritis, skin diseases and sinus problems, there were a large number who had a range of complaints which would nowadays be identified as forms of intercostal neuralgia, irritable bowel syndrome, acid reflux, diverticulitis, Crohn's disease or other predominantly gastrointestinal conditions often brought on by stress but which in the eighteenth and nineteenth centuries were diagnosed as hypochondriasis. This diagnosis often recognised a psychosomatic dimension. Sometimes the term 'valetudinarian' was used for these patients, as it was by Tobias Smollett when he described the Royal Mineral Water Hospital in Bath as 'that great hospital of the nation, frequented by all the valetudinarians whose lives are of consequence to the commonwealth'. There has been much debate about exactly what distinguishes hypochondriacs from valetudinarians – one pithy definition has it that whereas the former think they are always ill, the latter take great care to ensure they never are. However they were labelled, those with undue anxiety about the state of their health, usually centred around their bowels or intestines, formed a high proportion of those attracted to spas.

Hypochondria by its nature was an imprecise condition that tended to manifest itself in a general unspecified malaise. According to the American writer James Kirke Paulding, 'the most common infirmity which brings people to watering places is the disease of I don't know what.' For him, it was a peculiarly female affliction, which began with the sufferer complaining about 'the intolerable heat of the town' and fanning herself violently for several days. 'If this don't do, she begins to complain of weakness and want of appetite and spirits; and if this don't do, the doctor is called in, who, to get rid of a patient whose disorder he knows to be incurable, recommends a trip to the springs' (Chambers 2002: 76–7). The nature of spa treatments often exacerbated a sense of there being something wrong even when there was not because of the way that they tended to make you feel worse before they made you feel better. Augustus Granville described the typical progress of someone undergoing a cure at Bad Gastein:

> The patient experiences lowness of spirit or depression during the course of bathing and residence; at his departure, irritability, excitation, over-energy follow; in a month or two after his return home, languor and exhaustion succeed; and these are, in their turn, displaced after another month or so, by the conscious enjoyment of invigorated health. (Granville 2012: 89)

Granville was struck by the preponderance of hypochondriacs in the Continental spas through which he travelled. In Karlsbad, he found the most common *Kurgast* to be 'the despondent, dejected, misanthropic, fidgety, pusillanimous, irritable, outrageous, morose, sulky, weak-minded, whimsical, and often despairing hypochondriac' who was affected by 'continued indigestion, obstinate and unremitting gout, affections of the nerves of sympathy and the gastric region'. These 'unfortunate beings' were congregated in large numbers at the main drinking source, the *Sprudel*, every morning (Granville 2012: 113). His observations of the *Kurgäste* at

Wiesbaden prompted further reflection on this most common of all spa types:

> What a dreadful picture of human wretchedness the hypochondriac presents! He is sombre, thoughtful, or absent, in the midst of a laughing world. For ever brooding over his fate, his disease absorbs the whole of his attention. He disdains even the most trifling conversation with his fellow creatures, and flies from those ephemeral acquaintances which are so easily formed at watering-places, precisely because one cares little how soon afterwards they are forgotten. In fact, he would feel himself alone in the world, and never concern himself about those around him, did he not envy their healthy looks, their firmer muscles, and their sounder stomachs, which can sustain an indigestion with impunity. (Granville 2012: 186)

To some extent, the hypochondriacs who congregated in such large numbers in the spas of Europe throughout their golden age formed a buffer between the seriously ill patients and the idle pleasure seekers and provided a bridge between health and hedonism, desperation and decadence. They were in many ways the staple spa clients and for some observers they were the most authentic element in a company largely made up of charlatans and posers. An article in *Punch* in 1858 about those who resorted to Continental watering places concluded that 'the only honest portion are hypochondriacs' (Morgan 2014: 88).

Allied to the sense of profound ennui and melancholy that stays in spas induced, hypochondria exacerbated the tendency to develop a morbid introspection. This could manifest itself in an obsessive interest in one's bowel movements and urinary flow, as exemplified in the precise record of such matters kept by Michel de Montaigne on his travels through European spas in the mid-sixteenth century (see page 84). It could also prompt a more profound kind of literary reflection, as in the case of Alice James, who, having been diagnosed with hypochondria's close cousin 'hysteria' in 1884, travelled from the United States to England, where she spent the last six years of her short life (she died at the age of forty-three). She divided her time between London and Leamington Spa, whose waters had been prescribed for what English doctors re-diagnosed as 'gouty diathesis'. At Leamington she stayed in a boarding house, spending every morning in bed, getting up in the afternoon and apart from an occasional outing in a Bath chair, spending the rest of the day on a sofa, reading, writing and receiving occasional callers. It was there that she began to keep the diary for which she is best remembered. Her account of how and why she started it in 1889 combines images of thermal water (ejaculation, geyser) with a sense of the boredom and introspection of the long-term spa resident:

> I think if I can get into the habit of writing a little about what happens, or rather doesn't happen, I may lose a little of the sense of loneliness and desolation which abides with me. My circumstances allowing of nothing but the ejaculation of one-syllabled reflections, a written monologue by that most interesting being, *myself*, may have its yet to be discovered consolations. I shall at least have it all my own way and it may bring relief as an outlet to that geyser of emotions, sensations, speculations and reflections which ferments perpetually within my poor old carcass for its sins. (Strouse 1981: 274)

It is perhaps partly the intense introspection which comes with hypochondria that accounts for the fact that there has been so much writing about spas in the form of journals, letters and novels on the part of those staying in them. As in the case of Alice James, writing has been a form of therapy for those trapped in the stifling self-absorption induced by their enervating and oppressive atmosphere. Writers have also been drawn to spas as a subject by their fascinating cast of cosmopolitan characters, their beguiling fairy-tale quality and their intriguing interplay of health, hedonism and hypochondria.

The book that follows makes use of many of these rich literary sources, along with the author's own personal observations, to explore especially the hidden history of spas: the undercurrents and eruptions that mimicked their mysterious subterranean waters; the goings-on behind the façades of their elegant Biedermeier buildings and the closed doors of their underground treatment rooms; the secrets and shadows, self-made and imposed, that followed people around as inevitable companions in this strange enchanted, bewitched, artificial world of *der Kurschatten*.

CLASSICAL ORIGINS

Bathing in thermal mineral waters was practised by the most ancient human civilisations. Indeed, baths built around hot springs during the Minoan civilisation, which flourished on the islands in the Aegean Sea between 2700 and 1500 BC, are among the oldest archaeological remains in Europe. It is, however, from classical times that appreciation of both the healing power and the pleasure of this practice really dates. The ancient Greeks and Romans studied the properties of water, built baths and developed sophisticated rituals around bathing and drinking. They also first forged the association between spas and loose living and sexual shenanigans.

There was widespread belief among the ancient Greeks in the healing powers of natural spring water for animals as well as humans. It was coupled with veneration of what they regarded as a sacred element created and sustained by the gods. Temples known as *asclepieia*, staffed by priests and dedicated to Asclepius, the Greek god of medicine and healing, were erected near springs and doubled as worship shrines and healing places. One of the earliest, in existence from at least the sixth century BC, was situated at Epidaurus in a valley full of mineral springs at the foot of Mount Kynortion. People came to them both as pilgrims and patients. After taking a bath for ritual cleansing on arrival and making an offering to Asclepius or one of the other gods associated with healing, those seeking a cure were put to bed in dormitories and often sedated with opium. The dreams that they experienced in a trance-like state on their first night were interpreted by priests who prescribed appropriate treatment. Ideally, the god himself would appear in a dream to intervene, as he apparently did to a woman named Andromache desperate to have a child who had come to the *asclepeion* in Epidaurus in the mid-fourth century BC. According to a text on a relief sculpture now in the Archaeological Museum at Piraeus: 'She slept in the sanctuary and saw a dream. It seemed to her that a handsome boy lifted up her dress, and after that the god touched her belly with his hand. After the dream a son was born to Andromache from her husband Arybbas.'

Andromache is the first woman recorded coming to a spa because she wanted to have a child. The account of her dream suggests that she might perhaps also have been one of the earliest to experience *der Kurschatten*. Was the handsome boy who lifted up her skirt a figment of her imagination or was he indeed the one who gave her the son she had wanted? In her case, the dream was apparently enough to effect a cure. For others, the treatment prescribed at the *asclepieia* involved a mixture of bathing and drinking, physical exercise, copious bloodletting and surgery. A man suffering from pleurisy who presented himself at the *asclepeion* at Pergamon was told to lie on his side and covered with a mixture of ashes and wine, while a patient spitting blood was told to eat pine-cone seeds with honey. Much use was made of the healing tongues of dogs and snakes, as in another case recorded on a relief sculpture in Epidaurus:

> A man with a wound on his toe was healed by a serpent. He was in a terrible state when the temple servants transferred him and sat him on a seat. When sleep came upon him, a snake came out of the abaton [a rectangular portico near the temple] and healed the toe with its tongue. When the patient woke up and realised he was healed, he said that he had seen in his dream a handsome youth putting a drug upon his toe.

The 200 or more *asclepieia* established across ancient Greece took on several of the characteristics of later European spas. Originally sited beside mineral springs in remote areas of great natural beauty, they gradually grew to encompass not just a temple and baths but communal dormitories and dining halls, and often a theatre, gymnasium, library and hippodrome for chariot or horse races.

People resorted to the *asclepieia* out of a widespread belief that regular bathing not only aided personal cleanliness but also maintained the unity and harmony of body, mind and soul. Hippocrates, often regarded as the father of medicine, was almost certainly trained at the *asclepeion* on the island of Kos and his experience there may well have influenced his strong enthusiasm for hydrotherapy. Believing that good health was achieved through a perfect mingling of sunlight and water, he wrote a treatise on 'Airs, Waters and Places', which emphasised the superiority of natural springs over rainwater and other more stagnant sources such as lakes. He advocated immersion in both hot and cold water, the former being beneficial in the case of fevers and the latter for digestive and abdominal troubles. Hippocrates is associated with developing the idea that the key to good health lies in balancing the humours, as represented by the four bodily fluids of blood, black bile, yellow bile and phlegm. To achieve this balance, he recommended physical exercise, daily bathing and massage with fragrant oils. He was somewhat less enthusiastic about swilling down large quantities of neat mineral water, especially when it had a strong sulphur or iron content, and recommended always mixing water with wine before drinking it. He even recommended giving children watered-down wine rather than milk.

The Hippocratic Corpus, a collection of books written by Hippocrates and his disciples, laid down precise instructions as to which conditions to treat with baths:

Bathing suits pneumonia rather than ardent fevers, for it soothes the pain in the chest, brings up the sputum, eases respiration and removes heaviness in the head. Do not bathe those with loose or constipated bowels, or those who are liable to nausea, vomiting, or bleeding from the nose. (Phillips 1973: 84)

The Greek historian Herodotus was the first writer to observe and describe the curative properties of thermal waters. He recommended those suffering from a variety of ailments to drink and bathe in the waters for twenty-one days, a period that was to become the norm for many later spa cures. Archimedes made a significant contribution to hydrotherapy by showing how buoyancy and upward pressure make bodies weigh less in water, benefiting those with mobility problems. Asclepiades, a Greek physician who practised in Rome, took issue with Hippocrates about the humours while agreeing with him in prescribing liberal quantities of wine in addition to water. He believed that crucial to health were the tiny openings on the surface of the skin, which allowed fluids to pass in and out of the body. Disease was caused when they became blocked, constricted or too relaxed. He advocated bathing in both hot and cold water to open and close the pores and regulate the system. The idea that mineral traces from thermal waters pass through the skin into blood vessels and tissue continues to be held by advocates of spa medicine today. The last of the great Greek physician-philosophers, Galen, who was himself as a teenager apparently cured of a dangerous illness, probably smallpox, at the *asclepeion* in Pergamon, where he subsequently studied and practised, was the most enthusiastic of all about the therapeutic benefits of bathing in thermal mineral waters, which he recommended combining with opium consumption for maximum effect. He was responsible for one of the first, and most comprehensive, catalogues of the ills that it could cure, which included headaches, vertigo, deafness, epilepsy, apoplexy, poor sight, bronchitis, asthma, coughs, spitting of blood, colic, jaundice, hardness of the spleen, kidney stones, urinary complaints, fever, dropsy, leprosy, menstrual problems, melancholy 'and all other pestilences'.

As well as being the subject of serious medical and scientific analysis, the healing properties of thermal mineral waters played a central role in Greek mythology and religion. The seventy-five hot springs at Aidipsos (now called Edipsos and a popular spa resort) on the island of Evia were said to have been created by Hephaestus, the god of fire, who smote the rock with his hammer and brought forth steaming water from the bowels of the earth at the behest of Athena, the goddess of wisdom, so that her protégé, Hercules, could come and rest there after his labours. Hera, goddess of women, marriage and childbirth, is said to have advised Deucalion, son of Prometheus, and his wife Pyrrha, to immerse themselves in the waters there in order to bear plentiful and healthy children. They did so and produced two children, one of whom was the redoubtable Helen of Troy. Therma, on the island of Ikaria, developed as a healing centre in the fourth century BC on the basis of its highly radioactive waters and is still a popular spa resort today. It was named after the Greek word for heat. Hot sulphur springs in the pass of Thermopylae near the city of Lamia were seen as forming the entrance to Hades in Greek mythology. Homer added to the appeal of thermal waters for the Greeks by referencing them several times in his epic poem the *Odyssey*. The aches and pains of Odysseus's travels were eased by hot baths specially prepared for him by the sorceress Circe and by Queen Arete. He emerged from them 'looking more like a god than a man'.

Attitudes to bathing in thermal waters changed over the period of Greek civilisation. Early on, it was widely seen as a decadent and effeminate practice. This was to some extent the view of Homer and it was shared by Socrates who prided himself on taking only occasional cold baths. Cold baths and showers remained popular with the Greeks who agreed with Victorian public schoolmasters and muscular Christians that they were good for both body and soul. Gradually, a less austere view came to prevail, although the emphasis in the ancient Greek approach to bathing remained very much on its capacity to strengthen, improve and cultivate the human body rather than on its pleasurable aspects. Bathing was part of a regime of vigorous physical exercise. Indeed, baths took second place to the *gymnasia* and *palaestrae* (wrestling schools) and their primary purpose was often for athletes to wash off the dust and oil from their bodies after their exertions. A vigorous workout in the gymnasium was seen as an essential prelude to brief sessions in the hot tub and the steam or 'sweat' room. Baths constructed at Olympia around the middle of the fifth century BC were among the first exercise complexes incorporating swimming pools, heated tubs, saunas, steam, vapour and herbal baths as well as *gymnasia* and *palaestrae*.

Despite their supposed health-giving benefits, Greek baths were dirty, sweaty and sordid places. They were regularly used as urinals and became notorious haunts of violence and casual sex. Galen noted without any apparent disapproval of the practice, 'someone recently asked us why we piss cold in the baths, but outside hot, not understanding that the piss itself is lukewarm' (Mattern 2013: 20). He also wrote about an aggressive youth who visited a gymnasium to bathe and fought with another man over space on the massage table, an early indication of how spas bring out the worst in people. Evidence from vases and drawings suggests that both sexes bathed naked together in baths and were also naked for exercises and games in the *gymnasia*. Homosexuality was encouraged. The *palaestrae* provided opportunities for looking at and touching naked boys while wrestling with them. Aristophanes refers to men hanging around the *palaestrae* trying to seduce boys and in his comedy *The Birds*, a character who had met a handsome boy coming from his bath in the gymnasium is chided by his father: 'you neither spoke to him, nor kissed him, nor took him with you, nor ever once felt his balls.'

In several significant ways, ancient Greek attitudes established principles that were adopted by later European spas. They included the shift from religious veneration to an emphasis on the body beautiful and cheating age, while maintaining an element of ritual and mystery, and the associations with fecundity and sexual adventures. What the Greek baths lacked was sophistication and grandeur. They were essentially adjuncts to the gyms and not designed for lingering or wallowing in.

The Romans inherited the Greeks' enthusiasm for bathing in thermal waters but were less concerned about its benefits to the body and much more interested in its pleasurable and social aspects. For them it was first and foremost a leisure activity and a sensuous experience, often described with the Latin word *voluptas*, to be indulged in daily and communally. It is significant that while the Greeks preferred cold baths, or at least extolled their virtues, the Romans liked their water hot. It mattered little whether their baths were filled with water that was naturally thermal and mineral-rich or artificially heated. Enthusiasm for bathing, which grew steadily through the period of the empire, crossed the social classes and embraced servants and slaves as well as better-off members of society. It is not too much to call it an obsession and it has even been described as the nearest that the Romans had to a civic religion. Unlike the Greeks, the Romans did not swim in their baths but spent long periods simply sitting in them soaking up the heat. They knew that this was not particularly healthy but that did not deter them. As the text on the tombstone of an ex-slave in Rome dating from the first century AD put it: 'Wine, sex and baths ruin our bodies, but they are the stuff of life – wine, sex and baths.'

From the early second century BC the Romans were building baths across the lands they conquered and occupied. They took over many of the Greeks' healing centres based around natural hot springs, including Aidipsos (which they renamed Aedipsus) and Thermae, equipping them with substantial stone baths and ancillary buildings. The oldest known baths in Italy, the Sabian baths at Pompeii, which date back to the fourth century BC, were also inherited from the Greeks. By the time it was buried under volcanic lava following the eruption of Etna in AD 79, Pompeii had three large centrally located bathing complexes and a fourth sited just outside the city walls. The 'suburban baths', as they have been dubbed by archaeologists, are notorious for the sexually explicit murals, each individually numbered, which have been discovered high up on the wall of a changing room. They include depictions of two women, a threesome and a foursome all engaging in what Mary Beard describes as 'athletic sexual intercourse' (Beard 2009: 248). It is thought that these frescoes, of which there seem originally to have been twenty-four, may have served as a menu for the various services provided in the brothel upstairs, or have acted as a rather racy aide-memoire to help bathers find similarly numbered lockers below. Roman baths became notorious pick-up places and were regularly used for prostitution and sexual encounters. A line of graffiti on the wall of the suburban baths in Herculaneum records two satisfied customers: 'Apelles the mouse with his brother Dexter lovingly fucked two women twice.' A scribbled price list for 'nuts, drinks, hog's fat, bread, meat and sausage' at the same location indicates the amount of eating that took place in and around baths.

A similarly louche atmosphere pervaded Baiae, the earliest and most developed Roman spa town. First established around hot sulphurous springs in the active volcanic region on the north-west shore of the Gulf of Naples around 200 BC, it grew to become a favourite resort of the ultra-rich. Substantial bathing establishments were built over the next 400 years, of which the remains of some can still be seen on the hillside overlooking the modern town of Baia, although much of the original resort now lies submerged under the sea as a result of volcanic activity. Baiae was in many ways a prototype of the later European spa, not least in its mixture of health and hedonism. It attracted Romans who stayed for between fourteen and twenty-one days to take a cure and others who made much shorter visits for wild parties and drunken orgies. The poet Martial noted in the late first century AD that his friend Laevinia, a sober and virtuous wife when at home, ran off with a younger man when she visited its baths. Earlier in the century, Seneca the Younger had described Baiae as a resort of luxury and vice to be avoided at all costs. This did not stop him taking a property there. He wrote that staying there was like 'living in a café' with drunken people wandering along the shore and the 'lakes a-din with choral song'. He deplored the soft and effeminate practices of the bathers in getting a sweat up in the steam rooms when 'perspiration should follow only after toil' (Seneca 1917: 337–9). He also gave a graphic description of the noises he heard from the bathing establishment next to his apartment:

> Picture to yourself the assortment of sounds, which are strong enough to make me hate my very powers of hearing! When your strenuous gentleman, for example, is exercising himself by flourishing leaden weights; when he is working hard, or else pretends to be working hard, I can hear him grunt; and whenever he releases his imprisoned breath, I can hear him panting in wheezy and high-pitched tones. Or perhaps I notice some lazy fellow, content with a cheap rub-down, and hear the crack of the pummelled hand on his shoulder, varying in sound according as the hand is laid on flat or hollow. Then, perhaps, a professional comes along, shouting out the score; that is the finishing touch. Add to this the arresting of an occasional roysterer or pickpocket, the racket of the man who always likes to hear his own voice in the bathroom, or the enthusiast who plunges into the swimming-tank with unconscionable noise and splashing. Besides all those whose voices, if nothing else, are good, imagine the hair-plucker with his penetrating, shrill voice – for purposes of advertisement – continually giving it vent and never holding his tongue except when he is plucking the armpits and making his victim yell instead. Then the cake seller with his varied cries, the sausageman, the confectioner, and all the vendors of food hawking their wares, each with his own distinctive intonation. (Seneca 1917: 373)

Like the Greeks, the Romans gradually changed and softened their approach to bathing. Initially, it was seen primarily in utilitarian terms with the emphasis being on washing and getting clean. Through the period of the Roman Republic (from 509 BC to 27 BC) it became a regular part of urban life. In the subsequent imperial age, the focus switched to sociability, leisure and pleasure. This change had much to do with the patronage of emperors, several of whom were themselves enthusiastic bathers and built elaborate baths. Nero, emperor from AD 54 to 68, is said to have coined the memorable phrase '*sanitas per aquam*' (health through water) whose initial letters may possibly provide the origin of the modern word spa. He also commissioned the first bathing complex in Rome to include a *palaestra*. Commodus, emperor from 177 to 192, is said to have bathed seven or eight times a day. Perhaps this was in conscious reaction to his father, Marcus Aurelius, with whom he ruled jointly for three years, and who was emphatically not an enthusiast, writing 'What is bathing when you think of it? – oil, sweat, filth, greasy water, everything revolting.' Several historians and philosophers shared his disgust over their contemporaries' enthusiasm for bathing and saw it as a decadent, self-indulgent activity, which was all right for the effete Greeks but had the potential to sap the sturdy manliness of the Roman Empire. Tacitus, whose views were perhaps clouded by the fact that he lived over a very noisy bathing establishment, bracketed 'the lounge, the bath and the banquet' as vices that the conquering Romans brought to Britain and so 'seduced the hardy native inhabitants of the island'. Seneca complained during the early days of the empire that bathing was losing its primitive simplicity and becoming soft, pampered and licentious. In the Republican era, military heroes had washed their tired bodies 'under a filthy roof and on a very poor floor', but now 'the walls are shining with rare marbles, the vault is covered with rich gilding and Thasian marble, which at one time could only be admired in the rarest temples, today lines the pools where weak bodies, covered by sweat from the ovens, dive into' (Bradley 2012: 49). Pliny the Elder complained that the baths were too hot and weakened the physical as well as the moral fibre of the bathers. Moralists were concerned that the emphasis on hedonism, sensuousness and *voluptas* made the bath houses a byword for promiscuity and effectively turned several into brothels.

There was also concern about what would now be called health and safety issues. With no disinfectant, the water was often very contaminated, not least with human excrement. Not all baths had a supply of running water and considerable impurities built up. Bathers were not always very careful about their personal hygiene. Martial wrote of one woman: 'In order to craftily substitute for such a reek another odour, whenever she strips and enters the bath she is green with depilatory, or is hidden behind a plaster of chalk and vinegar, or is covered with three or four layers of sticky bean-flour' (Jackson 1988: 50). Baths were a breeding ground for bacteria and the run-off of hot thermal water, which concentrated in stagnant pools, provided a perfect habitat for malaria-bearing mosquitoes. It was not uncommon for people to faint in the baths, especially when the wood from boilers heating the water gave off too much smoke. Bathers often drank too much. Pliny the Elder complained about those who used the sweat chambers to raise a thirst and 'while still naked, they lift up huge vessels [of wine] as if to show off their strength and pour down the whole contents, vomiting up again immediately and then drink another jar.' Seneca complained of young people who 'drink on the threshold of the baths among the unclad bathers; even soak in wine and then immediately rub off the sweat which they have promoted by many glasses of wine' (Yegül 2010: 26). Critics were also concerned about the way that the baths encouraged casual sexual encounters. Successive attempts were made to outlaw mixed bathing – Hadrian promulgated a decree to this effect shortly after becoming emperor in AD 117 – but they do not seem to have proved very effective. Even when bathing was segregated, often by having women bathe in the morning and men in the afternoon, there were still plenty of opportunities for couplings in changing rooms and other more discreet venues in the bathing establishments. In his famous manual *Ars Amatoria* Ovid recommended baths as a convenient place of assignation for lovers.

Despite its many critics, bathing became ever more popular. By the middle of the fourth century AD, the city of Rome had over 850 bath houses, or *balnea*, and ten much grander and more luxurious bathing complexes built by successive emperors and known as *thermae*. The largest and most magnificent of these were the baths of Caracalla, which still stand as an evocative memorial to the Romans' love affair with bathing. Over 9,000 workers were employed in construction work, which began in AD 212, with the baths opening five years later. At their height, the baths of Caracalla are thought to have attracted between 6,000 and 8,000 bathers each day. They constituted a complete social centre with two libraries and *gymnasia*, concert and lecture halls and a variety of hot, cold and steam baths. Bathers would usually spend all afternoon there, often beginning with a workout in one of the *gymnasia*, before making their way to the central *frigidarium*, a vast hall equipped with four cold-water pools, flanked on one side by a huge swimming pool (*natatio*) and on the other by the *tepidarium*, a warm-water pool for relaxing the muscles and joints. This was followed by visits to the large circular *caldarium*, where the water temperature could reach 38 degrees Celsius (100 degrees Fahrenheit) the *laconicum*, providing dry heat, and the *sudatorium* (steam bath). Bathers would take a final dip in one of the cool pools in the *frigidarium* to close their pores.

This progression from cold through warm to hot and then back to cold again would be taken up by later spas – it can still be experienced in all its stages in the Friedrichsbad in Baden-Baden – as would the Romans' practice of applying perfumed oils and sweet-smelling unguents to their skins at the end of a session in the baths.

The Caracalla baths had their own hidden side in the shape of a vast underground 'city', which incorporated heating and drainage systems, a water-powered mill, bakery and laundry and also a huge temple to Mithras, the mysterious Indo-Iranian god who was seen as presiding over the waters. The Mithraeum, as it is known, survives today as a stark but imposing brick-walled vaulted building decorated with a fresco of the god and a marble block carved to represent a snake in the rocks, from which Mithras was supposedly born. The most striking feature of the bare cave-like chamber is a hole in the middle of the floor that archaeologists believe to be the *fossa sanguinis*, or hole of blood, over which a bull would have been sacrificed in the rite which was at the heart of the cult's worship. The existence and prominence of this religious temple at the heart of the baths complex suggests that, at least as far as the *thermae* were concerned, Roman bathing had a spiritual dimension and was not simply a matter of sociable self-indulgence.

At the height of their popularity, many Romans from across the social spectrum were spending several hours every day lazing around in the baths which doubled as social clubs, libraries and cafés. They tended to go there in the afternoon after a morning's work, a light lunch and a short siesta. Much business was done in the baths and some stayed on to have their evening meal there. There was relatively little interest in the therapeutic benefits of bathing, although in the mid-first century AD Pliny the Elder wrote about the benefits of mineral waters for curing a range of diseases affecting the liver, kidneys and digestive tract as well as for easing rheumatism and arthritis, and the physician Aulus Celsus did recommend the use of sweating rooms for fevers. Bathing was very much a public rather than a private experience with the sociability, noise, grand scale and sumptuous decoration of the baths all contributing to the sense of *voluptas*. Baths even came to be regarded as good places in which to die. Despite his distaste for their decadence, Seneca chose to end his life in AD 65 by taking poison, severing several veins and sitting in a warm bath where, according to Tacitus, he suffocated in its steam. He was almost certainly influenced by Epicurus, who after two weeks of pain from kidney stones, went into a hot bath and gulped down wine to bring about his own end, and by Tullius Marcellinus, who was troubled by chronic illness and, after fasting for several days, lay down in a very hot bath where he gradually expired, in Seneca's words '*non sine quadam voluptate*' (not without a certain pleasure).

The Romans took their enthusiasm for bathing in thermal water with them throughout their empire. The original Spa in Belgium was first mentioned by Pliny the Elder around AD 77: 'In Tongaria, a region of Gaul, there is a famous spring whose water sparkles with bubbles and has a distinct aftertaste of iron. The water is an excellent purgative; it cures tertiary fevers and dissipates kidney stones. When the water boils, it bubbles furiously and leaves behind a red residue.' Several of Europe's great spas were first established as bathing centres by Roman legionaries, many of whom came from the south of Italy and found the climate north of the Alps distinctly chilly. They enthusiastically embraced the places with naturally warm waters that they encountered on their marches and which eased their rheumatism. Among them were Vicus Calidus (literally 'the hot town', later Vichy), Aquae Aurelia (Baden-Baden), Aquae Cetiae (Baden bei Wien) where the legionaries built baths fed directly from the hot springs in the late first century AD, and Aquae Helveticae (Baden bei Zürich), which recent excavations suggest may have been the largest Roman spa complex north of the Alps.

Perhaps the best preserved and best known Roman baths are those in Aquae Sulis, now Bath, unique in Britain in having natural thermal waters, which emerge at a temperature of 45 degrees Celsius (113 degrees Fahrenheit). It is clear that the springs here were venerated long before the Romans came. Stone Age hunters seem to have made offerings to them as long ago as 8000 BC and Celtic tribes also threw coins into the hot springs. An inscription mentioning the emperor Vespasian indicates that the Romans had built baths fed directly from the hot springs by AD 76 and a larger bathing complex was developed later in the first century.

It is significant that the Romans dedicated the baths jointly to Sulis, the Celtic goddess almost certainly associated with the hot springs before they arrived, and Minerva, their own goddess of wisdom who also had strong associations with healing. Sulis Minerva became the composite deity presiding over the hot springs and a substantial colonnaded temple dedicated to her was built adjoining the baths.

Between the temple and the extensive bathing complex was the source of the hot springs, which was venerated as the sacred heart of Aquae Sulis. Referred to in inscriptions as a *locus religioni*, or sacred place, the bubbling pool of greenish steaming water, which can still be seen today, was walled off and enclosed. It was regarded as the dwelling place of the goddess and no bathing was allowed there.

Those visiting Aquae Sulis in its heyday could swim in the naturally hot waters, sweat in a steam bath or a dry room similar to a modern sauna, and then plunge into a cold pool or sit immersed up to the neck in a variety of hot and cold curative baths. They could experience supernatural power and divine presence, take part in religious rituals presided over by priests in the temple, and throw votive offerings into the water. Over 12,000 Roman coins spanning the period from the first to the fourth century AD have been recovered from the area around the sacred spring. Even more intriguingly, so have 130 curses written on small lead tablets. Addressed to Sulis Minerva by those who had been wronged, usually through theft, they ask the goddess to curse and bring misfortune on their assailants and indicate a darker side to the purpose of this early spa.

Aquae Sulis almost certainly suffered with the official adoption of Christianity in Britain, as happened throughout the Roman Empire, in the early fourth century. It seems briefly to have flourished again with the revival of paganism later that century. An altar erected at the time of this revival refers to the 'restoration of a holy place wrecked by insolent hands'. The baths' new lease of life was short-lived, however. Flooding and damage caused by an earthquake led to their abandonment before the Romans left Britain at the beginning of the fifth century. Stones from the disused temple were used in the building of a Benedictine monastery on the site in the late seventh century. By then the baths had long ceased fulfilling any recreational, healing or religious function, victims in part of the 'insolent hands' of Christians who were very uneasy about the Roman addiction to bathing in thermal waters.

Several of the early fathers of the church attacked bathing as a sybaritic and sensual activity bound up with the worship of false gods. Writing at the end of the second century, Clement of Alexandria suggested that of the four motives which led people to frequent baths – cleanliness, health, warmth and pleasure – only the first two were legitimate:

> We must not think of bathing for pleasure, because we must ruthlessly expel all unworthy pleasure. Women may take use of the bath for the sake of cleanliness and health; men, only for the sake of their health ... the motive of seeking warmth is scarcely urgent, since we can find relief from cold in other ways. The continued use of baths undermines a man's strength. (Bradley 2012: 57)

Clement's near contemporary, Tertullian, believed that the Roman baths were full of idols and evil spirits on account of being so often resorted to by those seeking initiation into pagan cults like that of Mithras:

> Unclean spirits do settle upon the waters, pretending to reproduce that primordial resting of the divine Spirit upon them: as witness shady springs and all sorts of unfrequented streams, pools in bathing places, and channels or storage tanks in houses, and those wells called snatching-wells – obviously they snatch by the violent action of a malignant spirit. (Evans 1964: 12–13)

The belief that baths were haunted with demons and tainted by pagan ritual informed much early Christian literature. According to one version of the apocryphal Acts of John, probably written in the fifth century, John the Evangelist went to a bath house in Ephesus to cast out the demon who haunted it, probably the goddess Artemis to whom it was dedicated. In another version of the same story, he confronted the son of the procurator of the baths who wanted to use them for an amorous adventure with a prostitute.

Christian rigorists fiercely opposed bathing and took a positive pride in going unwashed. The fourth century biblical scholar St Jerome opined that 'he who has once bathed in Christ has no need of a second bath'. St Diadochos of Photiki, a fifth-century ascetic, expressed his conviction that while it was not strange or sinful to take baths, 'to refrain from them out of self-control I regard as a sign of great restraint and determination. For then our body will not be debilitated by this self-indulgence in hot and steamy water; neither shall we be reminded of Adam's ignoble nakedness, and so have to cover ourselves with leaves as he did' (Bradley 2012: 58–9). Barsanuphius, a sixth-century Palestinian hermit, was prepared to countenance bathing at times of illness 'but if a man is healthy, it cossets and relaxes his body and conduces to lust' (Bradley 2012: 59). In 423, St Augustine of Hippo advised a community of nuns not to visit the baths more often than once a month, and then only in groups of at least three.

The early church even developed a theologically based opposition to bathing in the doctrine and practice of *alousia*, the state of being unwashed. Its followers, predominantly priests, monks and hermits in the eastern part of Christendom in the fourth and fifth centuries, held that grace and godliness could be achieved only by shunning bathing and ignoring personal appearance. It was reported with pride that St Anthony had never so much as washed his feet during his whole life. Relics of this attitude persisted well into the early Middle Ages in monasteries and among those dedicated to the religious life. The early English church historian Bede noted that the seventh-century Abbess Aebba of Coldingham only took a hot bath before the major Christian festivals such as Easter, Pentecost and Epiphany.

Officially, the church authorities did not prohibit bathing but they made very clear that Christians should bathe only occasionally, observing strict rules and regulations, and that they should definitely not enjoy the experience. Nude and mixed bathing were absolutely taboo. Ambrosius, Bishop of Milan, decreed that while it was just about acceptable for Christians to visit baths during the daytime, it was sinful to visit them at night. Although a blanket ban was never imposed, people were left in no doubt that bathing was at best a necessary evil that conferred no spiritual benefits. Any suggestion that bathing might be indulged in as a pleasurable and relaxing experience was severely squashed. For Pope Gregory the Great, baths existed 'for the needs of the body', not 'for the titillation of the mind and for sensuous pleasure'. Christians were warned off attending bath houses because of both the risk they posed to their immortal souls and the sort of people they might find there. It was not surprising, given this overwhelmingly negative propaganda about bathing, that early Christians generally smelled less sweet than their non-Christian neighbours.

On the whole, the churches of the East looked on the practice of bathing more favourably than those in the West. Perhaps this was simply because the hot climate made frequent washing in water rather more necessary and appealing. The Cappadocian fathers Basil of Caesarea and Gregory Nazianzen are both reported to have taken thermal baths. Bishop Sissinius, Patriarch of Constantinople in the 420s, proudly announced that he bathed twice a day. Although St John Chrysostom deplored mothers spoiling their daughters with worldly luxuries like baths, his followers apparently regularly frequented the baths at Constantinople. Macedonius, Patriarch of Constantinople from 496 to 511, is also said to have led his monks in frequent bathing sessions. It is noticeable that the Byzantine, Arabic and Turkish societies of the Eastern Mediterranean kept the bathing culture of the classical world going after it had declined and virtually disappeared in Western Europe. This was not so much due to the influence of Eastern Orthodox Christianity, however, as to the significant boost that the practice received in the early seventh century from the teaching of the prophet Muhammad. He enthusiastically recommended bathing in warm water and was especially keen on the use of steam and sweat baths on the grounds that their heat enhanced fertility and would encourage followers of the faith to multiply. When the conquering Muslim armies encountered Roman and Greek baths in Syria and Egypt later in the seventh century, they enthusiastically embraced the pleasures of the bathing culture. So developed the hammam, that distinctively Islamic version of the spa.

In the Christian West, by contrast, the bathing culture developed by the Romans was in marked decline from the late fifth century onwards and had all but disappeared by the end of the eighth century. Opposition from the churches and from Christian moralists and preachers undoubtedly helped to hasten the demise of the bath houses but probably more decisive were physical attacks on aqueducts from invading Germanic tribes and the general collapse of the economy and infrastructure that came with the weakening and disintegration of the Roman Empire. The aqueducts to Rome were cut by the invading Goths in 537, leading to the abandonment of the Caracalla baths and the other *thermae* and *balnae* around the city. Roman bathing culture may itself have been a cause of the empire's decline. Critics claimed that too many hot baths had led to a weakening of male testicles and a fall in sperm count and virility. Historians have suggested that many people may also have been adversely affected by lead poisoning from the aqueducts and pipes that carried water to their baths. Whether the ancient Romans did indeed effectively drown in their own thermal waters or not, there has never been a people so devoted to baths and bathing. Later spas would copy much from them, not least by often directly imitating the architecture and layout of their great *thermae*.

2

THE MIDDLE AGES – FROM HOLY WELLS TO STEW HOUSES

The nineteenth-century French historian, Jules Michelet, described the period from the mid-sixth to the mid-sixteenth centuries as 'a thousand years without a bath'. It is certainly true that through much of the Middle Ages there was little interest across Europe in bathing in thermal mineral waters. Ironically, given the strong Christian opposition to the practice, it was largely monks who kept going or revived some of the earlier classical thermal springs and gave them a new lease of life as holy wells possessing miraculous properties and associated with local saints or with the Virgin Mary. In the later medieval period, from the thirteenth century onwards, natural hot-water bathing was taken up again, inspired partly by the enthusiasm of those returning from the Crusades having enjoyed the hammams of the Middle East, and also by the relaxing of austere Christian rigour and the advent of Renaissance humanism with its respect for classical ideas and practices. Thermal baths continued to have a dubious reputation, however, being known as *seminaria venenata*, or seminaries of sex and sensuality. They became notorious not just for sexual activity and general debauchery but also for their poor standards of hygiene and almost certainly contributed directly to the plagues that ravaged late medieval Europe.

Several of the thermal spas first named and established by the Romans flourished as early medieval holy wells. The healing waters at Spa came to be associated with a local saint, Remaclus, a Benedictine missionary bishop who died around 673 after founding several monasteries in the Ardennes region. He reputedly possessed powers to purify fountains and generate springs. Some centuries after his death, healing miracles were recorded at the springs that he had supposedly blessed, including one in which a blind woman bathed her eyes and immediately regained her sight. A belief arose that any young woman who drank the waters of the Sauvenière spring and stood in an imprint of Remaclus's foot reputedly left on a stone nearby was assured of progeny and as a result many brides were taken there by their husbands. Building work at this spring in 1980 to renew the piping uncovered what appeared to be such an imprint and it can now be seen on the stone pavement surrounding the fountain. The transition from holy well to fully fledged spa is usually taken to have begun in 1326, when an ironmaster from nearby Liège who claimed to have been cured in its chalybeate springs set about developing it as a therapeutic resort. By 1351, so many visitors were coming to take the waters at Spa that a cure tax was imposed.

In Britain, the baths at Aquae Sulis, which had fallen into disrepair and neglect after the departure of the Romans, seem to have been at least partially reopened at some point by the Benedictine monks who founded a monastery adjacent to the old disused baths around 675. It is not clear quite when this happened, nor when the monks came up with the Anglo-Saxon term *Hat Bathu* (Hot Baths) from which Bath gets its name. There is little evidence of much use being made of the baths until the early twelfth century when John de Villula, Bishop of Bath and Wells from 1088 to 1122 and a physician as well as a priest, established Bath as a centre of healing by constructing three new baths for public use. They were administered by the Benedictine community at the nearby abbey. Despite remaining under monastic and ecclesiastical supervision, the baths acquired a reputation as places of debauchery and vice. In 1449, Bishop Beckington threatened with fire and excommunication those who bathed in them without proper clothing, word having reached him 'that the heavenly gift of warm and healing waters with which the City of Bath has been endowed from of old is turned into an abuse by the shamelessness of the people of that city'. Judging by subsequent similar pronouncements over the next couple of centuries, attempts to get bathers to cover up had little effect.

Other medieval spas had similar close links with local monasteries. Alsatian monks seem to have used the thermal waters at Aquae Aurelia (Baden-Baden) for therapeutic purposes from the mid-seventh century. The baths at Pfäfers were developed and administered by monks from the Benedictine Abbey at the top of the Tamina Gorge. They were responsible for looking after those who bathed in the thermal waters and seem to have been generous in providing for their needs – in 1504 sixty cartloads of wine were apparently somehow conveyed to the bottom of the gorge. Another famous spa had monastic origins. Premonstratensian monks from Teplá established a small community near the strongly sulphurous springs in the vicinity of the village of Auschowitz in Bohemia in 1341 and later started decanting the water into barrels, which they sold at a handsome profit. People came to drink from the Stinkquelle, or Stinking Spring, and those who felt that they had been cured by it left votive offerings to the Virgin Mary. As a result, the spring's name was changed to Marienquelle, giving the spa that would much later be established in a joint effort by the monastery's abbot and doctor its name of Marienbad (see page 133). According to its foundation legend, the nearby spa of Karlsbad owed its name to the fact that its springs were first discovered by the Holy Roman Emperor Charles IV while hunting in the Bohemian forests around 1350. One of his hounds fell into a pool of thermal water and, although initially scalded by the temperature of around 70 degrees Celsius (158 degrees Fahrenheit), seemed to enjoy the experience. The emperor followed his dog in and obtained relief from long-standing pain in one of his legs.

Some accounts of medieval bathing suggest that it was a masochistic practice informed by the fiercely ascetic tenets of Christian rigorism. A chronicle dating from 1113 describes those taking steam baths in wooden bath houses in Russia: 'They warm them to extreme heat, then undress, and, after anointing themselves with tallow, take young reeds and lash their bodies. They lash themselves so violently that they barely escape alive. Then they drench themselves with cold water and thus are revived. They think nothing of doing this every day and actually inflict such torture upon themselves voluntarily' (Allen 2004: 23). Other sources suggest a more gentle experience geared especially to the needs of the sick. An account from the late twelfth century describes the Knights of St John founding a hospital for lepers by the natural thermal springs that emerge from the bottom of Gellért Hill on the Buda side of the Danube, in what is now Budapest. St Elizabeth of Hungary, who lived from 1207 to 1231, is depicted in several paintings washing a sick man in a wooden bath tub there, and a French knight passing through Buda on the way back from a pilgrimage to the Holy Land around the same time wrote of the 'very fine warm baths' at the foot of the Gellért Hill.

Across Europe, when bathing did take place, it was not in grand and elaborate marble baths as favoured by the Romans but rather in wooden tubs, usually just big enough to accommodate two people. Medieval paintings suggest that they were often occupied by a man and a woman bathing naked, as in the coat of arms granted to the town of Baden bei Wien in 1480 by Emperor Frederick III (Plate 3). Later medieval bath houses opened far into the night, with meals being laid out on tables floating in the water, gambling taking place, walkways around the tubs allowing onlookers to feast their eyes on the bathers, and a repertoire of bawdy songs not dissimilar to later changing-room chants. Their somewhat louche atmosphere is well conveyed by the Italian humanist scholar Poggio Bracciolini's description of his visit to the baths in Baden bei Zürich in 1416. He reported that there were twenty-eight private baths, where 'men mix promiscuously' with women, surrounded by galleries. While bathing, men wore only a small apron while the women were clad in linen vests 'which are, however, slashed on the sides, so they neither cover the neck, the breasts, nor the arms of the wearers'. In addition, there were two public baths 'frequented by lower orders of people', where males and females were separated by a simple low railing: 'it is a droll sight to see the decrepit old women and blooming maidens exposing their charms to the profane eyes of men.'

Poggio was amazed that people would enter the baths two or three times a day and spend several hours in them at each session, amusing themselves by singing, drinking, dancing and playing musical instruments. There was much flirting. Men threw down coins 'which they direct to the fairer damsels. The ladies below stretch out their hands and spread their bath gowns to receive these gifts.' A large number of abbots, monks, friars and priests frequented the baths and 'forgetting the gravity of the profession, sometimes bathe with the ladies and adorn their hair with silken ribbons'. Poggio was entranced by the atmosphere, comparing the baths to the Garden of Eden and concluding that 'if pleasure can make a man happy, this place is certainly possessed of every requisite for the promotion of felicity ... For all people here concur in banishing sorrow, and courting mirth.' He had no doubt about Baden bei Zürich's contribution to the age-old role of spas in encouraging fertility:

I believe there are no baths in the world more efficacious in promoting the propagation of the human species. An immeasurable multitude of persons of all ranks repair to this place from the distance of 200 miles, not with a view of renewing their health, but of enjoying life. These baths are the general resort of lovers and their mistresses, of all, in short, who are fond of pleasure. Many ladies pretend to be sick, merely with a view of being sent for a cure to this watering place. You consequently see here a great number of handsome females without their husbands, and not protected by any male relations, but attended by a couple of maids and a manservant, or some elderly cousin, who is very easily imposed upon. And they come adorned with such costly apparel, that you would suppose they were coming to a wedding, rather than to a watering place. (Shepherd 1837: 81–7)

A similar atmosphere is conveyed in a miniature painted around 1470 by the Master of Anthony of Burgundy (Plate 2). Although illustrating a passage from a first-century Roman author about the baths of Sergius Orata and their use by Hannibal's troops, the scene is clearly modelled on a contemporary Flemish bath house. A man in courtly garb and a king are depicted observing nude men and women bathe and eat together in a row of wooden tubs, while two couples in the baths and a couple in an adjacent room fondle one another. The women wear elaborate veils and jewelled necklaces, suggesting that they are prostitutes. By the time of this painting, bath houses across Europe had become synonymous with brothels. They were known as 'stew houses', a term that, like the word 'bagnio', derived from the Italian *bagno*, served to designate both public baths and brothels. There are numerous descriptions of them in this latter role. The Italian scholar Bartolomeo Della Rocca encountered a prostitute in a steam bath in 1504 and after obtaining consent from her and her pimp, took the opportunity of inspecting her body in the interests of his research on human physiognomy. Some years later, another Italian writer, Tommaso Garzoni, deplored the way in which the once dignified profession of Roman bath attendant had become debased into that of pimp:

> Steam bath attendants [*stufaioli*] are engaged in washing, making sweat, applying cupping glasses, shaving body hair, and to clean all parts of the body in their baths, of which a great number can be found in Rome, Naples, Venice, Milan, Ferrara, Bologna, Lucca and in other Italian cities. Their vices concern the impurity of the flesh, because very few steam bath attendants are not pimps who rent rooms, blending inner dirt with external dirt in those baths, which are the cradle of a thousand shameful and dishonest carnal desires. (Garzoni 1996: 1322)

The Gellért Baths were developed by the Turks in the early sixteenth century and became known as the Atchik Ilidja, or Baths of the

Virgins. They were staffed by young girls who attended to bathers by massaging them with birch or oak-leaf brooms immersed in the hot water. Engravings show Budapest bath girls clad in skimpy aprons or diaphanous see-through dresses and holding the brooms and pails of water that were the tools of their trade. They did occasionally fulfil a loftier role. According to the *Bohemian Chronicle*, King Wenceslas III, a successor to the monarch immortalised in the well-known Christmas carol, was rescued from captivity at the hands of an evil usurper by a Budapest bath girl in the early fourteenth century.

As the bath houses effectively became the brothels of late medieval Europe, it was not uncommon for women to claim that they had become pregnant merely from bathing in water that had previously been used by a man, and the superstition arose that bath water was dangerously potent with 'frogges and other wormes' of fertility. Writing in the 1640s, the English scientist Sir Thomas Browne sought to scotch once and for all the idea, which he dated to the twelfth century but noted was still commonly held in his own time, that a woman could conceive in a bath, 'by attracting the sperm or seminal effluxion of a man admitted to bathe in some vicinity unto her'. He declared that it was impossible 'to fornicate at a distance and much offendeth the rules of physick, which say there is no generation without a joint emission, nor only a virtual, but corporal and carnal contact' (Browne 1888: 259).

By the end of the Middle Ages, bath houses had come not only to be associated with sexual immorality, gambling, theft and drunkenness but also to be seen as breeding grounds for contagious diseases. An outbreak of a particularly virulent and unpleasant strain of syphilis across Western Europe in the late 1490s, thought by some scholars to have been brought over from the New World by Columbus and by others to have been spread by the 50,000 troops who had occupied Naples in 1495 under the French king Charles VIII returning to their various homes across the Continent, led to strenuous efforts to clean up bath houses and stop mixed bathing. The effect of this new puritanism can be seen in a 1496 woodcut by Albrecht Dürer which shows a male-only bath; he also made a drawing the same year of a female-only bath (Plate 4). This was probably a topical reference, as communal baths in his own home town of Nuremberg were closed down that year in an attempt to halt the spread of the syphilis epidemic. His engraving shows four men lounging in an open-air bath house listening to two musicians. All have noticeably rippling muscles, although a rather more obese figure sits on the right-hand side downing a flagon of beer. On the other side, a rather languorous figure, thought to be Dürer himself, leans against a wooden post from which protrudes a tap that looks for all the world like a penis. Maybe this is a less than subtle reference to the reputation of baths as places for homosexual hook-ups.

The early sixteenth century saw several attempts by European monarchs to tackle the scourge of the stew houses. Francis I ordered most of France's bath houses to be demolished in 1538 and slashed the number in Paris from twenty-six to just two. Henry VIII banned mixed bathing in England's bath houses in 1546 and closed down several notorious stew houses in London. Somewhat ironically, just as the secular authorities were attempting to clean up Europe's bath houses, a development at the very heart of the Roman Catholic Church was reaffirming their traditionally rather risqué and racy image. One of the most bizarre and well- hidden secrets of the Vatican is the so-called pornographic heated bathroom, officially known as the Stufetta del Bibbiena, which was specially decorated by Raphael for Cardinal Bibbiena in 1516. The frescoes on the walls illustrate the erotic adventures of Venus and Cupid, which Bibbiena, a writer of comedies who served as treasurer to Pope Leo X, enjoyed as he lounged in his hot tub. The Vatican has long been somewhat embarrassed about this small room which is located in the Pope's private residence and it is very much off-limits to visitors. Several of the frescoes have been painted over, including a depiction of Vulcan attempting to rape Minerva, but among those surviving is one showing Pan leaving the cover of some bushes with a giant erection.

If the Stufetta del Bibbiena suggests a lingering love-affair on the part of the late medieval Catholic Church with the more hedonistic side of bathing in thermal water, the outlook of the Protestant Reformers on this, as on so much else, could not have been more different. Together with the rise in scientific rationalism and the development of the modern medical profession that came in its wake, the Reformation swung the emphasis from hedonism to health and helped give birth to the modern spa as a carefully regulated therapeutic establishment.

3

THE SIXTEENTH AND SEVENTEENTH CENTURIES – THE BIRTH OF THE MODERN MEDICAL SPA

The sixteenth century saw the birth of the modern concept of the spa as first and foremost a therapeutic facility curing illness and promoting health. This had much to do with the rise of the medical profession across Europe and the replacement of religious superstition by science-based evidence, trends that owed much to the new humanist scholarship and the influence of the Reformation. Shorn of their miraculous powers and associations, thermal mineral springs were carefully measured and classified according to their chemical composition. Their waters were tamed and controlled, funnelled through pipes and conducted to drinking halls and bath houses where they were provided for patients in carefully regulated quantities. Treatises written by qualified doctors included detailed chemical analyses of the contents of individual springs and sources, precise lists of the particular conditions that they could cure, and careful prescriptions of the appropriate daily regime for those undergoing treatments, with almost every hour accounted for. In this new, distinctly puritanical regime, drinking cures assumed at least as much importance as bathing. While they became increasingly fashionable thanks to royal and aristocratic patronage, spas never completely shook off the seedy reputation of the medieval stew houses but the accent, officially at least, was now firmly on health rather than hedonism.

Medical treatises on the benefits of thermal mineral waters had begun to appear in the late Middle Ages. One of the first to be written since classical times was *De balneis et thermis naturalibus omnibus Italiae* by Michele Savonarola. Although written in 1440, it was not published until 1531. As its title suggests, it covered natural thermal waters across Italy but it focused especially on those around Abano near Padua, where Savonarola practised as a physician, and which he recommended especially for treating skin diseases. Abano Terme remains a major spa specialising in *fango* or mud-based therapies today. Savonarola largely followed the ancient theory of bodily humours propounded by Hippocrates. A more up-to-date and scientific approach was displayed in a number of works published in the early sixteenth century. The earliest known book in German on the benefits of spa cures, *Ein Traktat der Badenfahrt* (Treatise on Spa Travels), was published in 1511. Written by Wolfgang Winterperger, who practised as a doctor in Krems, it described the therapeutic effects of several thermal waters, notably the Frauenbad and Herzogbad in Baden bei Wien. The first scientific study of the Karlsbad waters appeared in 1522 under the title *Tractatus de thermis Caroli IV Imperatoris*. Its author, Václav Payer, especially emphasised the importance of the drinking cure. The first detailed treatise on the waters of Baden-Baden was written following a visit there in 1526 by Theophrastus von Hohenheim, a Swiss physician, alchemist and astrologer with strong Protestant Anabaptist sympathies who took the name Paracelsus. In 1535, he turned his attention to the baths at Pfäfers, which he likened to Purgatory but commended for their effectiveness in cleaning the body of virtually every ill that might assail it. He specialised in the cure of syphilis and suggested that both drinking from and bathing in the Baden-Baden and Pfäfers thermal waters would relieve it and other diseases. His enthusiastic endorsement of spa treatments combined Protestant piety with a strong preference for natural remedies over drugs: 'So that sick people may be cured, the Lord has ruled in His creation that more strength be found in springs than in learned prescriptions' (Wechsberg 1979: 51). Several prominent humanists afflicted with syphilis duly took themselves off to Baden-Baden while the leading Swiss Reformer, Huldrych Zwingli, was persuaded to subject himself to the more forbidding atmosphere of the Pfäfers baths.

It was not just Protestant physicians who championed spas. In 1559, Gilbert Lymborgh, personal physician to the prince-bishop of Liège, wrote a treatise on the fountains of the Ardennes, which was translated into Latin, Spanish and Italian. This work played a key role in putting Spa on the map as a major cure resort for people from across Europe. Spa's reputation was further enhanced by a visit from Agostino, court physician to the English king Henry VIII, who was said to have been the first doctor to use its waters to treat rheumatism. In 1571 Andrea Bacci, a medical writer based in Rome, published *De Thermis*, an influential work on the therapeutic benefits of thermal waters. The publication of a pioneering scientific study of the sources at Vichy in 1605 led directly to the construction of the first thermal establishment in the town complete with baths and douches.

The advocacy of medics was also important in the development of British spas. Bath's credibility as a serious medical spa owed much to the work of Dr William Turner, a prominent English Protestant who studied medicine and theology at Cambridge. Pursuing a joint medical and clerical career, he became physician to the young King Edward VI's uncle and protector, the Duke of Somerset, and was installed as Dean of Bath and Wells in 1551. During the reign of the Catholic Queen Mary, he went into exile on the Continent, visiting and studying spas in northern Italy, Switzerland and Germany. His resulting book, *The Book of the Natures and Properties as well of the baths in England as of other baths in Germany and Italy*, was first published in 1561 following his return to England to resume his post as Dean of Bath and Wells under Elizabeth I. It listed no fewer than eighty-nine disorders that could be cured by bathing in thermal waters like those at Bath, among them piles, migraine, sciatica, worms in the belly, palsy, failure to menstruate, hectic flushes, premature ejaculation, forgetfulness, deafness, pimples, 'the scratch', 'old sores and blotches' and 'weakness of any member'. Turner advised drinking mineral water 'to scour the inside of the body', beginning with five cups of water every morning and gradually rising to twenty at the height of the cure. He also anticipated the nineteenth-century pioneers of hydrotherapy, Vincent Priessnitz and Sebastian Kneipp, by advocating the use of jets of water directed at specific parts of the body. This therapy was introduced at Bath in 1631 using special buckets with holes in the bottom.

William Turner's book covered ten therapeutic bathing resorts in Continental Europe but only one, Bath, in the British Isles. He noted that he was the first to write on this subject in English and that 'very few in times past have been by the advise [sic] of physicians sent unto these baths'. He castigated his countrymen for showing so little enthusiasm for bathing in mineral waters and so lightly regarding 'such high and excellent gifts of Almighty God'. He deplored the fact that while large sums of money were spent in England on cockfighting, tennis courts, banqueting and pageants, nothing was spent on baths and bathing. Like other Protestants, he saw natural thermal waters as a gift from God to be valued and treated with reverence and respect. He counselled those embarking on a cure: 'After you have confessed yourself before Almighty God, and to such as you have offended, in the name of God, take counsel with some learned physician who is sent of God, and not of some self-made idol, who is sent of himself.' His insistence on the importance of consulting a doctor was accompanied by a strong emphasis on a careful, well-regulated regime while taking the waters. His book recommended a hygienic approach to bathing with regular cleaning of the baths and a strict segregation of the sexes, unlike the 'beastly filthiness' that prevailed in Bath where 'contrary both unto the law of God and of man', male and female bathers were allowed 'to go together like unreasonable beasts to the destruction of both body and soul' (Lennard 1931: 3–4). Successive bishops of Bath and Wells followed his lead in promoting Bath's thermal waters as a God-given blessing to be used soberly and reverently for healing purposes only and not for licentious lounging about. In 1559, an episcopal decree laid down that anyone who had reached puberty must wear a robe while bathing.

In 1596, Dr Timothy Bright, who was personal physician to Elizabeth I, described Harrogate, where a chalybeate spring had been discovered in 1571 and which became the first resort in England to offer a cure based on drinking natural mineral water, as a 'spa' – or 'spaw', as he spelled it. This is the first recorded use of the term in English to denote a place with healing waters. He used it because Harrogate's waters tasted similar to those that he had sampled at the resort of that name in the Ardennes. The word was brought into wider currency following a visit to Spa around 1620 by two English doctors, Sir William Paddy and Dr Richard Andrews. They applied its name to all those places possessing natural mineral springs to which people resorted to drink or bathe for therapeutic purposes. Prominent among the early English spas was Buxton, whose waters were commended in a treatise written by a Welsh doctor, John Jones, in 1572, as especially efficacious for 'women that by reason of over much moisture, or contrary distemperature be unapt to conceive and weak men that be unfruitful'. He suggested that treatment with Buxton water also relieved haemorrhoids and piles and that 'for them that are given to wind it much availeth'. Together with liver and stomach complaints brought on by over-indulgence, infertility, piles and flatulence were to remain among the most commonly cited conditions amenable to treatment by a course of taking the waters. But there was virtually no limit to the list of ailments, both psychological and physical, susceptible to cure by this means. An analysis of the Tewit Well, a particularly iron-rich spring at Harrogate, by Dr Edmund Deane, a prominent York physician, in 1626 concluded that its waters killed worms in children, cooled the kidneys and bladder, and 'purged the blood of choleric, phlegmatic and melancholic humours. It cheereth and reviveth the spirits, strengtheneth the stomach, causeth a good and quick appetite and furthereth digestion' (Jennings 1981: 5).

Overall, these medical treatises emphasised drinking over bathing cures, while acknowledging a therapeutic role for both. The doctors who wrote them, and who increasingly took on the supervision of the early spas, advocated substantial exposure to their waters, both internally and externally. They regularly prescribed several litres of water to be drunk daily, usually in the early morning, and several hours of immersion in a bath. People coming to Karlsbad for a cure had been generally very reluctant to drink too much water because they were afraid that its strong mineral content would petrify inside them. This was not a wholly silly idea – even now there are warnings that drinking from some of its springs will increase the risk of kidney stones forming. However, a month-long drinking cure introduced there in 1520 prescribed eighteen glasses of the evil-tasting water on the first day, rising to forty glasses later on. An abacus-like device called a *Trinkuhr* (drink clock) was developed so that patients could keep count of their intake. Immersion in the baths was also prescribed at a level that would later be regarded as excessive and positively dangerous. It was not uncommon in Karlsbad for those taking a cure to be required to remain in the water for up to ten hours a day. Their skin became very chapped as a result, leading the baths to be described as *Hautfresser* (skin eaters). William Turner noted that at Baden bei Zürich the curative benefits of the thermal waters were only felt by those who spent four hours in the baths every morning and a further three in the afternoon, while for women seeking to cure their barrenness daily immersion for nine hours was recommended. On the whole, patients in British spas underwent a much less intensive regime than those on the Continent. Bathers in Bath were recommended to spend only one or two hours a day in the waters. Cures could last anything between three weeks and two months; anything less was unlikely to yield much in the way of benefits.

If medical endorsement was crucial to the development of Europe's spas, so also was royal and aristocratic patronage. Emperor Ferdinand I significantly enhanced the status and prosperity of Baden bei Wien in 1531 when he granted it the right to charge an entrance fee of two pfennigs to the bath houses which had been built over two springs. Spa's appeal as a resort for the fashionable was considerably boosted by visits in the 1570s from King Henry III of France. Karlsbad, which already claimed to be a royal foundation (see page 67), gained further kudos in 1630 from a well-publicised visit by Albrecht von Wallenstein, supreme commander of the forces of the Habsburg emperor during the Thirty Years' War. He came for a three-week cure to alleviate his gout, bringing with him fifteen oxen, ninety lambs, sixty-three barrels of beer and sixty-three buckets of wine, just in case the local supplies proved inadequate.

Royal patronage was especially important to the English spas. Buxton's fame was enhanced by visits from Mary Queen of Scots, who was let out of her imprisonment to go there five times between 1573 and 1584 and claimed to have derived much benefit from the baths. Her cousin, Elizabeth I, is not recorded as having undertaken any spa cures, although her reaction on learning that her courtier and favourite, the Earl of Leicester, was planning to take the waters in Buxton suggests that she did have an interest in the subject. She recommended that he be put on a severe diet and be given 'for his drink one twentieth of a part of a pint of wine to comfort his stomach, and as much of St Anne's sacred water as he lusteth to drink' (Lennard 1931: 9). Bath benefited from being visited three times in the early seventeenth century by Anne of Denmark, wife of James I, in an attempt to cure her dropsy (oedema). She bathed in a small rectangular bath that had been constructed in 1597 for the exclusive use of women. Following her visits, it was named the Queen's Bath.

Tunbridge Wells benefited considerably from aristocratic and royal patronage. The curative properties of its waters were supposedly first discovered in 1606 by Lord North, who had already taken the waters at Spa in an unsuccessful effort to repair the ravages of life at Court. Seeing a rust-coloured pool of water as he was riding through a 'barren heath' on the Kent and Sussex borderland, he took a swig and found that it tasted very like the Spa water. A sample that he took back to London was analysed by doctors who declared that it possessed curative properties. North himself returned to Tunbridge Wells to take the waters the following year. He found them more beneficial than Continental waters, which had the added disadvantage of being expensive to reach and 'inconvenient to religion'. Many English people objected to going to Catholic Europe to take a cure, and indeed the government was so worried that Spa had become a centre of seditious Catholic opposition to the Protestant English monarchy that an act of 1571 proscribed travel there without a special passport and official authorisation.

Queen Henrietta Maria, wife of Charles I, came to Tunbridge Wells for a six-week period of recuperation in 1630 following the birth of her son, the future Charles II. In the absence of any permanent buildings around the springs, the royal entourage camped in tents on the common. The first medical treatise on the Tunbridge Wells waters, entitled *The Queens Welles*, was published in 1632. Its author, Dr Lodwick Rowzee, recommended that they be drunk an hour or so after sunrise, and accompanied by caraway comforts 'to correct the flatulence'. He also suggested that 'after you have taken your full quantity, it will do well to walk up and down, and to compose yourself to mirth with the rest of the company; for those who look to reap the benefit by Tunbridge, must turn away all cares and melancholy' (Cunningham 2005: 19). To assist people in their promenading, a cobbled walkway to the principal spring was constructed in the 1630s, with an upper walk across the common being added later. There were further royal visits in the later seventeenth century. Charles II came several times, making a six-week stay with his court in 1663, as did his brother, James, and his niece, Anne. In 1698, while she was queen, Anne visited Tunbridge Wells with her son and heir, William, Duke of Gloucester, who suffered from hydrocephalus. He stumbled and fell badly while playing soldiers with other children on the rough cobbles of the walkway. Anne gave money for the path to be properly paved and was annoyed to find on a visit the following year that no paving had been laid. She departed promptly, never to return, ordering a superintendent to ensure that the work was carried out. The new paved walkway opened in 1700, and became known as the Pantiles. It remains a prominent feature of the town today.

Bath, too, attracted royal visitors. In 1663, Charles II brought his wife, Catherine of Braganza, there in the hope that immersion in its waters might help her become pregnant. In the event, all she came away with was a nasty skin disease. Mary of Modena, wife of James II, spent several weeks in 1687 bathing every morning in the Cross Bath in an effort to improve her chances of providing her husband with his much-wanted male heir. The birth the following year of Prince James, who was destined never to succeed to the throne but rather to become the Old Pretender following his father's deposition in favour of a Protestant succession, was attributed to the effect of the Bath waters. An elaborate cross erected in the Cross Bath in thanks for his birth later became the target for Protestant vandalism.

The combined effects of medical and royal endorsement helped to clean up the image of spas and bathing places across Europe but they did not entirely efface their reputation as glorified brothels. Successive attempts to outlaw mixed bathing and to make long ankle-length white linen bathing robes compulsory for men and women were not always successful. An imperial edict in 1626 outlawing nude bathing and establishing separate bath houses for men and women at Baden-Baden was overruled by the town councillors on the grounds that it would ruin business and damage the spa's prosperity.

Two well-known paintings suggest that baths continued to have a rather racy reputation throughout the sixteenth century. *The Fountain of Youth*, painted by Lucas Cranach in 1546, depicts haggard and overweight ladies entering a swimming pool and emerging lithe and pert at the other side, to dine, dance and disappear behind bushes with lusty male partners (Plate 5). Hans Bock's depiction of the baths at Louèche in Switzerland in 1597 shows men and women bathing naked in an outdoor pool. While some are involved in serious and solitary pursuits, such as reading a book or playing a musical instrument, others are clearly engaged in amatory adventures (Plate 6).

The atmosphere of the emerging spas of Europe is well caught in the letters and diaries of the many writers who frequented them for a cure. Few were more obsessively concerned about their own health than the French essayist Michel de Montaigne, who toured European spas between June 1580 and November 1581 in an effort to break up the kidney stones that were giving him excruciating pain. His travel journal reads like a clinical case history with particularly detailed accounts of his urinary and bowel movements, which were recorded in minute detail. There is also much about flatulence. He went first to Plombières in eastern France where he noted that those with syphilis were excluded from the baths and prostitutes were forbidden to come within 100 paces of them: 'Singular modesty is observed here; and yet it is indecent for the men to go in otherwise than quite naked except for a little pair of drawers, and the women except for a shift.' He noted that it was customary to bathe two or three times a day and drink a glass or two of water while in the bath. The locals considered Montaigne very odd for drinking nine glasses of water daily. At his next port of call, Baden bei Zürich, he was somewhat alarmed to find people being bled so heavily while bathing 'that I have sometimes seen the public baths look like pure blood'. He was particularly enamoured of the waters of the Bernabò spring at La Villa in Italy where he stayed for a total of seventy-four days. Having found that they were very efficacious in removing red pimples on the face, 'a fact I carefully note as a service I owe to a very virtuous lady in France' (presumably his wife?), he set about monitoring exactly what the waters produced in terms of sweat, stools and urine and was much exercised when the 'count of what I had urinated did not match with what I had drunk'. An extract from his diary over three successive days in August 1581 is typically graphic:

On the 16th I went to the women's bath, where I had not yet been, in order to be separate and alone. I stayed there an hour at most and sweated moderately. My urine was natural; no gravel at all. After dinner my urine came turbid and red, and at sunset it was bloody.

On the 17th I found this same bath more temperate. I sweated very little. The urine rather turbid, with a little gravel; my colour a sort of yellow pallor.

On the 18th I stayed two hours in the aforesaid bath. I felt I know not what heaviness in the kidneys. My bowels were reasonably loose. From the very first day I felt full of wind, and my bowels rumbling. I can easily believe that this effect is characteristic of these waters, because the other time I bathed I clearly perceived that they brought on the flatulence in this way. (Montaigne 1958: 1016)

Succeeding days provide similarly detailed and precise accounts of urinary excretions and bowel movements until at last there is this triumphant entry:

On the 24th, in the morning, I pushed down a stone that stopped in the passage. I remained from that moment until dinner time without urinating, in order to increase my desire to do so. Then I got my stone out, not without pain and bleeding, both before and after: as deep and long as a pine nut, but as thick as a bean at one end, and having, to tell the truth, exactly the shape of a prick. It was a very fortunate thing for me to be able to get it out. I have never ejected one comparable in size to this one. (Montaigne 1958: 1018)

Although Montaigne obtained relief from his kidney stones, he came away from his intensive round of Europe's spas with several new ailments, including toothache, headaches and eye troubles, all of which he blamed on the waters. It is something of a relief to turn from his morbid self-obsession to the observations of two English travellers who visited Baden bei Zürich a decade or so later without any desire to record their bowel movements. Following his stay in 1592, Fynes Moryson noted his impression of the baths:

> Men, women, monks and nuns sit all together in the same water, parted with boards, but so as that they may mutually speak and touch, and it is a rule here to shun all sadness, neither is any jealousy admitted for a naked touch. The water is so clear as that a penny may be seen in the bottom, and because melancholy must be avoided, they recreate themselves with many sports, while they sit in the water; namely at cards, and with casting up and catching little stones, to which purpose they have a little table swimming upon the water, upon which sometimes they do likewise eat. (Moryson 1825: 315)

Thomas Coryate came away from his visit to Baden bei Zürich in 1608 with a similar impression. He noted that the clientele consisted of 'gentlemen of great worth that repaired thither partly for infirmity's sake and partly for mere pleasure and recreation' and was somewhat surprised to see married women bathing naked with men who were not their husbands, 'and not only talking and familiarly discoursing but also sporting after a very pleasant and merry manner'.

> Here also I saw many passing fair young ladies and gentlewomen naked in the baths with their wooers and favourites in the same ... Many of these young ladies had the hair of their head very curiously plaited in locks and they wore certain pretty garlands upon their heads made of fragrant and odoriferous flowers. A spectacle exceeding amorous. (Strachan 1962: 73–4)

Pierre Bergeron, a French visitor to Spa in 1619, was impressed by its medical benefits and its amorous atmosphere. He seems to have swallowed copious draughts of propaganda as well as of water, enthusing that the springs could 'extenuate phlegm; remove obstructions in the liver, spleen, and the alimentary canal; dispel inflammations; comfort and strengthen the stomach and the nerves; purge wateriness and the peccant humours of choler and melancholy' in addition to having 'laxative and diuretic' properties and the almost obligatory added attribute of 'rendering women fecund'. An early and shrewd observer of the way that spas developed more hedonistic attractions to help 'banish all care, anxiety and melancholy' among those engaged in the serious business of taking the waters, he noted that 'from this follow all kinds of games and pleasures, concerts, dances, ballets, feasts, tilting at the ring, love affairs, serenades, philosophical discussions, and buffooneries.' Bergeron was struck by how a stay in Spa seemed to lead many *curistes* who came without their spouses to forget old loves and kindle new passions. This was not always conducive to a completely successful cure. A gentleman might repair his ravaged liver but pick up a new venereal disease or two, while those ladies who had hoped that the waters would aid their fecundity might become pregnant rather more quickly than they had anticipated (Bergeron 1875: 165, 183, 190).

The diarist Samuel Pepys, who visited several English spas in the 1660s, concentrated on writing about his own experience of taking the waters and the effect that they had on him. He drank five glasses from the well at Barnet in July 1664 and noted that the woman dispensing the water 'would have had me drink three more, but I could not, my belly being full'. He was much pleased by the vigorous effect on his bladder movements on the way home but had a 'mighty sweat' in the night 'till I melted almost to water' (Pepys 2003: 404). Despite this not altogether satisfactory experience, he returned the following month and again in 1667 to drink more water from the Barnet wells and in the latter year he also downed four pints from Epsom's famous saline springs.

The amatory possibilities presented by a spa cure were described in several poems written in and about Tunbridge Wells in the 1670s. This ballad of *c.*1678 gives an indication of the way that the town marketed itself to the fairer sex:

> You ladies who in loose body'd gown
> Forsake the sneaking city,
> And in whole shoals come tumbling down,
> Foul, foolish, fair or witty.
> Some for the scurvy, some the gout
> And some for love's disease,
> Know that these wells drive all ill out,
> And cure what e'er you please;
> They powerfully break the stone,
> And heal congestive lungs;
> They'll quicken your conception,
> If you can hold your tongue. (Cunningham 2005: 8)

In 1674, John Wilmot, the Second Earl of Rochester, a well-known libertine and courtier of Charles II, summed up the waters' best-known properties even more graphically:

> For here walk Cuff and Kick,
> With brawny back and legs and potent prick,
> Who more substantially will cure thy wife,
> And on her half-dead womb bestow new life.
> From these the waters get the reputation
> Of good assistants unto generation. (Vieth 1968: 79)

During his stay in Tunbridge Wells, Wilmot overheard a childless woman telling another that 'I'm informed these wells will make a barren woman as fruitful as a cony warren.' His overall impression of the spa was not very complimentary. He found the 'Company' affected, tedious and seedy, describing the well as 'the rendezvous of fools, buffoons, and praters, cuckolds, whores, citizens, their wives and daughters' (Vieth 1968: 73). Having failed to take his prescribed dose of water because the sight of everyone there made him 'purge and spew', he removed himself to the upper walk 'where a new scene of foppery began':

A tribe of curates, priests, canonical elves,
Fit company for none besides themselves,
Were got together. Each his distemper told,
Scurvy, stone, strangury; some were so bold
To charge the spleen to be their misery,
And on that wise disease brought infamy. (Vieth 1968: 75)

The journals of Madame de Sévigné, the French aristocrat who took a cure in Vichy to alleviate severe rheumatism in her hands just two years after Wilmot went to Tunbridge Wells, give a very different impression of spa life. She took her cure seriously and followed her doctor's advice to eat only boiled or roasted meat, shun anything fatty, avoid all alcohol except the occasional glass of white wine as least harmful to the digestion, and above all take care of her emotions as well as her body. He had told her, 'Tranquillity of the passions is the most important requisite for maintaining a good functioning of the body while taking the waters. That is why all affairs of importance and passions of the heart which destabilise the spirit are prejudicial to recovering health' (de Bennetot 1966: 19–20). She dutifully went to the source at 6 a.m. every day and bravely faced a regime which she found very unpleasant –'Oh, these waters are nasty'– on more than one occasion vomiting up her morning's intake. She found the routine of spa life exceedingly boring, with the morning spent simply in promenading, taking the waters and discussing their effect with other *curistes*, a very light lunch, the afternoon devoted to resting and playing cards, a light supper in the evening and bed at 10 p.m. The dullness was only alleviated by visits to the baths, which she described as 'a good enough rehearsal for Purgatory. One is completely naked in a little underground place where one finds a tube of hot water which a woman directs on you where you wish. This state where one keeps on scarcely a fig leaf of clothing is something quite humiliating' (de Bennetot 1966: 41).

Others made even more apocalyptic comparisons. A visitor to the King's Bath in Bath saw 'young and old, rich and poor, blind and lame, diseased and sound, English and French, boys and girls, one with another, peep up in their caps and appear so nakedly and fearfully in their uncouth postures as would put one in mind of the Resurrection' (Rolls 2012: 18). Willem Schellinks, a Dutch artist who visited Bath in 1662, expressed concern about the close proximity of baths for horses and for humans and also about the number of people who felt faint after sitting for several hours in the hot water. He noted that they were given hot wine boiled with sugar and herbs to revive them. In 1668, Samuel Pepys recorded his unease at entering the Cross Bath at 4 a.m.: 'me thinks it cannot be clean to have so many bodies together in the same water.' After two hours in the bath, he was 'carried away, wrapped in a sheet and home to bed, sweating for an hour'. He had found the water exceptionally hot and was impressed by the number of men and women who seemed to spend hours there every day 'that cannot but be parboiled and look like Creatures of the Bath' (Morshead 1926: 488–9). Ned Ward, a satirist who wrote about Bath at the very end of the seventeenth century, was alarmed by the appearance of the bath attendants employed by bathers to 'scrub their putrefying carcasses like racehorses'. Making the familiar comparison with the Underworld, he described them as 'infernal emissaries' because 'by their scorbutick carcasses and lacker'd hides, you would think they had laid pickling a century of years in the Stygian lake.'

Like earlier visitors to Continental spas, Ward was struck by the amorous atmosphere of the baths at Bath, writing of the mixed Cross Bath:

> Here is performed all the wanton dalliance imaginable; celebrated beauties, panting breasts and curious shapes, almost exposed to public view; languishing eyes, darting killing glances, tempting amorous postures, attended by soft music, enough to provoke a vestal to forbidden pleasure, captivate a saint and charm a Jove. The vigorous sparks present the ladies with several antick postures, as sailing on their backs, then embracing the element, sink in a rapture and by accidental design thrust an outstretched arm; but where the water concealed, so ought my pen. The spectators in the galleries please their roving fancies with this lady's face, another's eyes, a third's heavy breasts and profound air. In one corner stood an old lecher whose years bespoke him not less than three score and ten, making love to a young lady not exceeding fourteen. (Rotherham 2014: 13)

Although the baths at Bath clearly provided much titillation for those who ventured into them, standards of safety and hygiene continued to leave much to be desired. There were several cases of drowning in the early seventeenth century and the water was often contaminated by the presence of animal carcasses as well as human bodies. In 1676, Bath Corporation was impelled to pass a series of by-laws prohibiting bathers from smoking, singing bawdy songs and making such disturbances as 'rendered the baths like so many bear gardens'.

One of the last and most thorough chroniclers of English spas in the seventeenth century was Celia Fiennes, who visited twenty-seven active mineral water springs around the country between 1685 and 1700, carefully noting what she saw of both their medical and their social side. They included places such as Canterbury, Wigan, Hackney and Dulwich, which once had thriving mineral water wells but later ceased to be spas. Not surprisingly, given that it was well on the way to overtaking Tunbridge Wells as the most popular and fashionable English watering place, she was particularly interested in Bath, which she found confined and stuffy with a prevalent atmosphere of disease. She gave a detailed description of the baths, which men entered clad in drawers and waistcoats made of a fine yellow canvas and women in stiff garments made of the same material 'with great sleeves like a parson's gown ... the water fills it up so that your shape is not seen.' Bathers sat up to their necks in the water, with the seats in the middle of the baths being occupied by men and those round the sides by ladies. Entering one of the baths herself, Celia Fiennes needed someone to guide her 'for the water is so strong it will quickly tumble you down' but once inside there were rings to hold on to. In the King's Bath she saw the treatment recommended by Dr Turner being put into practice with people being 'pumped at' on their legs for lameness or on their heads for palsy: 'I saw one pumped, they put on a broad brimmed hat with the crown cut out, so as the brims cast off the water from the face. One of the men guides the pumps – they have twopence I think for 100 pumps. The water is scalding hot out of the pump' (Morris 1982: 45). Willem Schellinks had also been intrigued by the number of pump strokes, as he called them, being administered to people in the baths – as many as 1,800 in some cases. Celia Fiennes was relieved to discover that the baths were regularly emptied and refilled. When new water was added, there was a white scum, which attendants had to skim off before anyone entered as it caused heat rashes and pimples. She also found that in general modesty and decorum seemed to prevail around the baths, with a serjeant patrolling the galleries to ensure that order was observed and rude behaviour punished. Her remarks suggest that matters of hygiene and discipline had at last been taken in hand by the end of the century.

The other leading English spas did not receive quite such a vote of confidence from Celia Fiennes. She found Buxton very overcrowded – guests in the boarding house where she stayed had to sleep three to a bed – and was disappointed that there seemed to be no provision for regularly cleaning the baths or replenishing the water, which was so cold that 'it made me shake'. As in Bath, the waters in the Buxton baths had a strong current: 'You must have a guide who swims with you; you may stand in some place and hold by a chain and the water is not above the neck, but in other parts very deep and strong and it will turn you down' (Morris 1982: 108). In Harrogate, the smell from the 'sulphur or stinking spaw' was 'so very strong and offensive that I could not force my horse near the well' and 'it has an additional offensiveness like carrion or a jakes [toilet].' She congratulated herself on managing to drink a quart of its evil-smelling waters 'and hold them to be a good sort of purge if you can hold your breath so as to drink them down' (Morris 1982: 93). Harrogate's sulphur well had a generally unsavoury reputation. Some years before Celia Fiennes's visit, Michael Stanhope, a local doctor, observed that it was used for bathing and drinking predominantly by the 'vulgar sort' in an effort to treat their skin diseases. It was especially resorted to by lepers 'whose putrid rags lie scattered up and down, and it is to be doubted whether they do not wash their sores and cleanse their besmeared clouts where divers after dip their cups to drink' (Jennings 1981: 6).

Despite the many scare stories about their unsavoury aspects, spas across Europe were becoming established by the end of the seventeenth century as places to go to cure all manner of diseases by drinking and bathing in their natural mineral waters. There was a good deal of hype around them, as in this doggerel verse extolling the merits of Buxton:

Old men's numb'd joints new vigour here acquire,
In frozen nerves this water kindleth fire.
Hither the cripples halt, some help to find,
Run hence, their crutches unthanked left behind.
The barren wife here meets her husband's love,
With such success she straight doth mother prove.

There was also a fair amount of cynicism, as evidenced by an anonymous comment made in 1661 about the rapid growth of spas:

> Let them find out some strange water, some unheard-of Spring. It is an easy matter to discolour or alter the taste of it in some measure. Report strange cures that it hath done. *Beget a superstitious opinion of it.* Good fellowship shall uphold it, and the neighbouring towns shall all swear for it. (Rattue 2001: 122)

4

THE EIGHTEENTH CENTURY –
THE EMERGENCE OF BATH AS
THE MODEL SPA

It was in the eighteenth century that Europe's spas came into their own as elegant resorts for the well-heeled upper and middle classes, drawn initially by the therapeutic benefits of taking the waters and increasingly also by the diversions offered and the chance to mix with the rich and titled. Spas became the pre-eminent places in which to be seen and to socialise. They developed a distinct architectural landscape in which the bath house was joined by a pump room, for taking the waters and promenading, and assembly rooms, for socialising, gambling, dancing and concerts. Typically constructed in neoclassical style, these buildings were situated in attractive parks with lawns, rare trees and lakes, adding to the atmosphere of elegance and relaxation. A complex set of rules and strict etiquette governed the social life of spas during the 'season', which could extend from March to November but was more usually confined to the months from May to September. During this period 'the Company', as the patrons were known, forsook the noise and the stench of cities for the clean air and healing waters of these semi-rural oases, which were promoted as Utopian paradises.

The English were in the van of these developments, taking to the waters more enthusiastically and in greater numbers than their Continental neighbours. Bath established itself in the first half of the eighteenth century as both the most elegant and the most popular

European spa, with John Wood laying out its crescents, circles and squares in Palladian style and Richard 'Beau' Nash establishing the complex etiquette that governed the social and recreational life of the Company. It became the model for Continental spas, notably Spa, Baden bei Wien and Baden bei Zürich, which developed in a similar way in the latter half of the century. They followed Bath's lead in establishing a daily regime for guests, which began with the serious business of drinking and bathing in the waters, continued with morning and afternoon promenades and social gatherings to exchange gossip, and concluded with balls, gambling, concerts and theatrical performances in the evening.

Initially, it was the health-giving properties of their waters that gave these places their *raison d'être* and attracted visitors. 'Mineral water has never been so much of an issue as in this century' wrote Théophile de Bordeu, official superintendent of the mineral waters of France, in 1775. Spa cures involving precisely prescribed drinking and bathing regimes became increasingly popular throughout the eighteenth century. They were enthusiastically promoted by doctors who took up residence at the spas and established flourishing practices there. The emphasis shifted from the earlier detailed chemical analyses carried out by the pioneer spa physicians to a more general and less scientific focus on detoxing and wellness, not dissimilar to that found in spas today. This approach was well calculated to appeal to a growing leisured and moneyed class suffering the effects of over-indulgence, obesity and an increasingly sedentary lifestyle. Many physicians saw spa practice as a lucrative and undemanding career and the greedy quack, attached to a fashionable watering place and attracting credulous patients through shameless puffing and self-promotion, became a familiar figure in eighteenth-century poetry and fiction.

The growing popularity of spas was a direct consequence of the emergence during this period of what would now be called health tourism. The Enlightenment brought a new emphasis across Europe, and especially in Britain, on environment and on the benefits of travel for healing the body as well as cultivating the mind. Increasing pollution, noise and stench in cities fostered a search among those who could afford it for places to escape to, if only temporarily, where the air was fresher, the water cleaner and the atmosphere calmer. Health tourism was a key aspect of the Grand Tour on which so many aristocratic and well-off men and women embarked in the eighteenth century. Indeed, for many, a curative stay in one or more spas became an almost obligatory part of it. It was the English spas, and especially Bath, that picked up the benefit, becoming the first resorts to which people travelled as much for a change of scene as for other purposes.

Underlying this spa craze was a widespread preoccupation with ill health. As the social and medical historian Roy Porter observed, 'as the eighteenth century wore on all manner of men, great and small, rich and less rich, calibrated their lives according to their pains' (Porter and Rousseau 1998: 93). Several factors combined to bring this about, among them a decline of religious belief with its attitude of acceptance of suffering, the influence of Enlightenment ideas encouraging an introspective focus on the self, and the hype promulgated by a medical profession that was at its most entrepreneurial and unscrupulous before the tighter regulations that were to govern it in the nineteenth century. Illness came to be regarded as a state of mind as much as a process of nature and, indeed, almost as the normal human condition, as expressed by Alexander Pope when he referred to 'this long *Disease*, my life'. Once again, the English were in the forefront of this trend, producing an impressive number of prominent hypochondriacs who devoted much of their literary talent to worrying obsessively about their ailments, real and imagined, and chronicling their symptoms in precise detail. They included Samuel Johnson, William Cowper, Horace Walpole, Henry Fielding, Tobias Smollett, Jeremy Bentham, Sydney Smith and Samuel Taylor Coleridge.

One illness dominated this national narrative and drove many of its sufferers to seek spa cures. As used in the eighteenth century, when it was perhaps applied more frequently than any other medical term, the word *gout* covered a multitude of conditions, including what would now be diagnosed as rheumatism, arthritis, irritable bowel syndrome, diverticular disease, chronic gastroenteritis and myalgic encephalomyelitis/chronic fatigue syndrome. In its classic and simplest form, it was brought on by a high concentration of uric acid in the blood and manifested itself in painful swelling of joints in the extremities of the body, especially the big toe. This was quite often accompanied by kidney stones, the development of a more widespread arthritic condition and other more general and unspecific symptoms of malaise. Gout was caused by over-indulgence, especially in alcohol and rich and fatty foods, and its prevalence in this period can be directly related to several specific triggers. A treaty with Portugal in 1703 led to a huge rise in the English consumption of port (of which it was not unusual for people to be drinking a bottle a day), Madeira and other fortified wines. The ill effects of these beverages were exacerbated by the use of lead in the casks in which they were stored and the widespread adulteration of alcohol with lead-based additives. The agricultural revolution in the early decades of the eighteenth century led to a rise in meat consumption, especially of beef and mutton. The increasing adoption of carriages meant that the upper classes were walking less and leading more sedentary lifestyles. A vicious circle of over-consumption and lack of exercise produced a similar epidemic to the rise of Type 2 diabetes and other obesity-related diseases today.

Gout was regarded as a disease of the affluent, 'the patrician malady' as Porter dubbed it. It became highly fashionable, especially among literary figures, to the extent that you could hardly make it as an essayist, poet or novelist if you did not suffer from it or some other similar malady that took on obsessive proportions and became a main theme in your writings. Closely related to gout were intestinal disturbances and bowel movements, which similarly became something of a national obsession. In Porter's words, 'popular physiology' in the eighteenth century 'attended to evacuations no less than to appetites' (Porter 1993: 601). Flatulence and farting are favourite topics in the era's novels and poems. Leading doctors were agreed that spas were the perfect places to cure the mixture of digestive and nervous symptoms displayed by those suffering from gout and the closely related condition of hypochondria. When Erasmus Darwin was consulted in 1787 by a woman suffering from a burning sensation in her stomach, vomiting, indigestion and nervous weakness, he had no hesitation in recommending that 'a journey to Bath might be of service to you' (Darwin 2012: 273).

Bath established itself as Britain's premier health resort first and foremost on the basis of its claim to be able to diagnose and treat these conditions. Its appeal to the gout-ridden and hypochondriacal, preoccupied by the state of their bowels, is well illustrated in Christopher Anstey's satirical and hugely popular poem, *The New Bath Guide*, first published in 1766. Anstey himself was a classic example of the eighteenth-century spa enthusiast. Following a period of depression aggravated by ill health after the death of a beloved sister in 1760, he was advised to take the waters at Bath. He was so impressed by their therapeutic effects that he returned annually and eventually decided to settle there permanently, taking a house in the newly built Royal Crescent. The hero of his poem, Thomas B-r-d, troubled by loose bowels and almost constant flatulence, comes to Bath with his sister, his cousin and their maid seeking a cure for their various distempers and graphically describes the doctor's verdict after their first consultation:

> He determin'd our cases, at length, (G-d preserve us!)
> I'm bilious, I find, and the women are nervous;
> Their systems relax'd, and all turn'd topsy-turvy,
> With hypochondriacs, obstructions, and scurvy;
> And these are distempers he must know the whole on,
> For he talked of the peritoneum and colon,
> Of phlegmatic humours oppressing the women,
> From foeculent matter that swells the abdomen;
> But the noise I have heard in my bowels, like thunder,
> Is aflatus, I find, in my left hypochonder. (Anstey 1770: 12–13)

Like other spas, Bath benefited from having a royal imprimatur. Having forsaken Tunbridge Wells, Queen Anne, who like so many of her subjects suffered from a range of complaints in the region of her abdomen, stomach and bowels, made several visits there in 1702 and 1703, increasing its appeal as a fashionable resort. By 1715, more than 8,000 visitors were arriving annually for the main autumn season which lasted from late October until Christmas. A slightly less fashionable spring season ran from late January until early June. Later on in the eighteenth century, the two became merged and Bath was 'on heat' for much of the year with the season effectively lasting from autumn to early summer. In this respect, it was very different from most Continental spas, which had their main season in the summer. Guests stayed for anything from two weeks to two months, drinking and bathing in the thermal mineral waters daily under the direction of one of the many doctors who set up practices in the town. Bath established a particular reputation for its 'gout doctors'. The best known, George Cheyne, made a lucrative career out of treating his affluent patients while also seeking to cure himself of the ravages brought on by a lifetime of gluttony, obesity and anxiety. He authored a trio of bestselling medical manuals which directly addressed the main illnesses, and imagined illnesses, that brought people to Bath. *Observations Concerning the Nature and Due Method of Treating the Gout* (1720) distinguished three types of gout: the most usually diagnosed form, with swellings of the joints at the extremities; 'nervous or flying gout', characterised by a biliousness which he observed in many of his Bath patients; and 'windy gout ... which is nothing but a *hypochondriacal* or *hysterical* symptom.' Alongside drinking and bathing in the Bath waters, the treatments he recommended for these conditions included blistering and bleeding and, in cases of gouty stomachs, purgatives and laxatives which 'may bring on the piles ... but will discharge the gout of the guts'. He also had a word of encouragement for sufferers from the patrician malady: 'Gouty persons', he observed, 'are people of good natural parts, large feeders and long-lived.' *An Essay of Health and Long Life* (1724) dispensed advice on plain living, avoiding excess, reducing meat intake, forswearing alcohol in favour of milk, and advocated a 'diet drink' made up of juniper berries, Seville oranges and honey. Cheyne's third bestseller, *The English Malady: A Treatise on Nervous Diseases of all Kinds* (1733), was a hypochondriac's handbook, mixing social snobbishness with medical mumbo-jumbo and arguing that it was only the elite who were 'privileged' to suffer from nervous ailments.

Among the well-known figures who came to Bath primarily to seek a cure for gout were William Pitt the Elder, who took a house in the newly built Circus in 1768, the year he retired as prime minister, and Horace Walpole, who dubbed it 'the Great National Hospital for Incurables'. Although most of the spa doctors shamelessly talked up the water's curative powers, some of the more honest acknowledged that often the main benefits to patients came from other aspects of their stay. For William Stevenson, a physician who wrote extensively on gout and practised briefly in Bath in the late 1770s,

> The merit of the Bath waters consists all in *negatives*. To drink them, you must leave the noise, hurry, and complexity of business; you must leave your crapulary debauch, your bottles, your women; nay more, you must leave your affected, hypocritical self, for your best resemblance, the *childhood of Nature*, and then drink the waters of life at Bath! (Stevenson 1779: 117)

John Penrose, an Anglican clergyman who took a cure in Bath in 1766, came to a similar view, noting that 'many other causes may possibly concur towards it, though here the waters run away with the credit' (Penrose 1983: 94). *The New Bath Guide* also struck a sceptical note about the miracle-cure claims about the water, with Thomas B-r-d's cousin Jenny declaring:

> She was shock'd that so many should come
> To be Doctor'd to Death, such a Distance from Home,
> At a Place where they tell you that Water alone
> Can cure all Distempers that ever were known. (Anstey 1770: 28)

There were other serious conditions which do seem to have responded to treatment with the Bath waters. Patients with skin diseases accounted for around 15 per cent of admissions to the Bath General Hospital, which opened as a charitable institution in 1742 and later became known as the Royal Mineral Water Hospital. One of the most badly affected was a fifteen-year-old girl, Mary Tompkins, who had been sent to St Bartholomew's Hospital in London with suspected leprosy but discharged as incurable. She came for in-patient treatment at Bath in 1763 under the care of Dr Thomas Oliver (best known as the inventor of the Bath Oliver biscuit) who wrote:

> I never saw so bad a leprous case. The girl's skin was almost universally covered with large, thick, hard, dry scabs of a dark brown colour. These brown scabs were specked with white shining silver scales which gave her countenance a very shocking appearance. The clefts between the scabs were wide and deep so that her skin resembled the bark of a tree. (Rolls 2012: 113)

Oliver prescribed a treatment of drinking a pint of mineral water daily and bathing twice weekly, together with the application of ointment made from a mixture of tar and oil extracted from the hooves of oxen, and a medicine containing mercury, antimony and sarsaparilla. Mary Tompkins' condition steadily improved and she was able to leave hospital after seven months 'perfectly cleansed'. A hospital exclusively designed for those suffering from leprosy was established in the 1750s alongside the Lepers' Bath which had existed since the twelfth century.

Another area in which Bath's doctors specialised was the treatment of lead poisoning. Around 8 per cent of the patients admitted to the general hospital were diagnosed with *colica Pictonum*, paralysis arising from chronic lead poisoning. Surviving records enable a comparison to be made between the success rates in the treatment of patients with this condition at Bath and at the general hospital in Exeter between 1762 and 1767. Whereas 73 per cent of the 285 patients treated in Exeter for *colica Pictonum* over this period were either cured or underwent a substantial improvement in their condition, the comparable figure for the 281 treated in Bath (who included eighty referred from Exeter after unsuccessful treatment there) was 93 per cent. Clinical trials conducted in the late 1980s by Dr Audrey Heywood, a Bristol-based doctor specialising in renal medicine, confirmed the benefits of using Bath's thermal waters in the treatment of chronic lead poisoning and the alleviation of kidney and liver disease. Unusually among modern British medical practitioners, she concluded that there is clear scientific evidence to justify the claims of Bath's enthusiastic eighteenth-century physicians that 'Bath spa therapy could be recognised as an effective cure, not merely a pleasant experience' (Heywood 1990: 101).

While the medical side of the spa continued to be important to those who came to Bath, especially with serious illnesses, for a growing number of visitors the social aspects and diversions came to be its main lure and attraction. This was particularly the case with the affluent and literary-inclined gouty valetudinarians. In a series of flirtatious letters written by Alexander Pope during a stay there in 1714, ostensibly to cure his gout, he scarcely mentions the waters but notes rather how 'I have slid, I cannot tell how, into all the amusements of this place; my whole day is shared by the pump-assemblies, the walks, the chocolate houses, raffling shops, plays, medleys &c' (Pope 1847: 328). Daniel Defoe, visiting in the early 1720s, reported that Bath had become 'the resort of the sound, rather than the sick; the bathing is made more a sport and diversion, than a physical prescription for health; and the town is taken up in raffling, gaming, visiting and, in a word, all sorts of gallantry and levity' (Defoe 1928, 2: 34). He found much the same at Tunbridge Wells, noting that 'the coming to the Wells to drink the water is a mere matter of custom; some drink, more do not, and few drink physically: But company and diversion is in short the main business of the place; and those people who have nothing to do anywhere else, seem to be the only people who have any thing to do at Tunbridge' (Defoe 1928, 2: 126). Often, it was the combination of the waters and the diversions that drew those in low spirits to spas, as in the case of Lady Orange, one of the 'Bath characters' described in a book of that title, who 'came hither to console herself on the loss of her first husband with Bath waters and *cassino* [a card game]' (Warner 1807: 59).

The most successful spas were those that merged the medical and the social and provided a range of attractions and diversions to alleviate the frankly dull and depressing business of taking their waters. In Bath's case this was achieved largely through the efforts of Richard 'Beau' Nash, who arrived in the town in 1704 at the age of twenty-nine. Nash had had a rackety early career, dropping out of Oxford University, probably to escape a woman, briefly holding a commission in the Guards and then practising unsuccessfully as a barrister in London. It was his addiction to gambling that took him to Bath. Within a few months of his arrival, this 'fastidious Welsh opportunist', as he has been dubbed, found himself as aide-de-camp to the Master of Ceremonies, Captain Webster, who superintended the social life of the spa. Webster was killed in a duel over a gambling debt in 1705 and Nash took over his role, remaining in post until his death in 1761. Extravagantly dressed with fancy waistcoat and black wig topped by a jewelled cream beaver hat, he became a familiar sight around the town and there was virtually no area of its social life that he did not personally supervise. He imposed rigorous rules of etiquette on all who came to take the waters, meeting new arrivals to judge whether they were suitable to join the select Company, matching ladies with appropriate dancing partners at each ball, enforcing a dress code for men and women, brokering marriages, escorting unaccompanied wives and regulating gambling by attempting to restrain compulsive gamblers and warning players against risky games and known cardsharps. Duelling and the carrying of swords by men were prohibited, begging was suppressed and Nash personally supervised the cleaning, paving and lighting of the streets.

Although Nash is rightly credited with improving Bath's moral and physical atmosphere and giving it an air of genteel respectability, he himself epitomised the more hedonistic and seedy side of spa life. Despite styling himself guardian of 'the young, the gay and the heedless fair' and warning young ladies of the designs of philanderers and fortune hunters, he entertained a string of mistresses in his house on Saw Close, near the Theatre Royal. He also remained a compulsive gambler, accumulating severe debts and eventually being forced to move in with one of his mistresses, Juliana Popjoy. When he subsequently left her for another woman, she was so distraught that she is said to have spent her remaining days living in a large hollowed-out tree.

Nash was also Master of Ceremonies at Tunbridge Wells from 1735. He was able to combine the two roles because the peak season there was in July and August, which was between seasons in Bath. In his first year at Tunbridge Wells, he attracted 900 'ladies and gentlemen of quality' there, including seven dukes and duchesses, fifty-three marquesses, earls and barons, sixteen knights and three MPs. The prime minister, Robert Walpole, came for three days to visit his mistress who was taking a cure there. While Tunbridge Wells claimed to have all that Bath offered in the way of gambling, concerts and balls, it also boasted 'amusements of a higher nature, equally calculated for the diversion and improvement of the serious and reflecting part of the Company'. In particular, it extolled the intellectual but cheerful atmosphere of its Circulating Library, Bookshop (where, unusually, ladies were admitted) and Coffee House:

> Here divines and philosophers, Deists and Christians, Whigs and Tories, Scotch and English, debate without anger, dispute with politeness, and judge with candour: while everyone has an opportunity to display the excellency of his taste, the depth of his erudition, and the greatness of his capacity, in all kinds of polite literature, and in every branch of human knowledge.
> (Burr 1766: 127)

Tunbridge Wells's intellectual appeal proved a less effective draw than Bath's combination of gout doctors and social snobbery. Even though it was closer to London and more attractively situated on its rocky heathland than the low-lying Somerset town, Tunbridge Wells never came near to challenging Bath's role as the most popular and fashionable English spa and the brand leader in early eighteenth-century Europe. What gave Bath its edge was a combination of its concentration of medical experts and facilities, its exceptionally elegant classical architectural layout and the daily regime established by Nash, which became the model for spas across the Continent.

Life for the Company revolved around a series of regular and prescribed rituals. The day began early with guests being carried from their lodgings in sedan chairs at around 6 a.m. to one of the bath houses, having followed medical advice to first evacuate their bowels and bladders. After immersing themselves in the steaming water for a couple of hours or so, they dressed and gathered in the Pump Room, built in 1706, to take their statutory three glasses of water, a much reduced intake from the eight to ten pints that had been prescribed daily in the seventeenth century. The Pump Room was substantially extended in 1751–2, with large windows put in to afford a good view of those wallowing in the adjoining open-air King's Bath, as described by Anstey in his *New Bath Guide*:

> Oh 'twas pretty to see them all put on their flannels,
> And then take the waters like so many spaniels:
> And though all the while it grew hotter and hotter
> They swam, just as if they were hunting an otter. (Anstey
>   1770: 38)

Following breakfast at a coffee house or in the Assembly Rooms, built in 1709 and extended in 1730, several of the Company attended a daily service at 11 a.m. or noon in the nearby abbey as much for social as spiritual benefit. Most then returned to the Pump Room to mingle or promenaded along the Gravel Walks. Dinner, the main meal of the day, was taken at 3 p.m. or 4 p.m., followed by a further visit to the Pump Room, more promenading and tea in the Assembly Rooms, often accompanied by the card games faro and hazard, gambling with dice and roly-poly, a forerunner of roulette. Attempts to curb gambling by increasing taxes on the purchase of playing cards and dice and putting legal limits on the sums that could be won or lost in a single session failed to dent the Company's enthusiasm for these and other games of chance. The evening was given over to more card playing and entertainments. A typical week's programme during the season included dress balls on Monday and Friday, less formal cotillion balls on Tuesday and Thursday, a subscription concert on Wednesday and a visit to the theatre on Saturday. The formal balls generally took place in either the 'Old' or 'Lower' Assembly Rooms near the baths, or the 'New' or 'Upper' Assembly Rooms constructed in 1771 near the Circus, and fell into two distinct halves. The first part of the evening, which began around 6 p.m., was given over to French dances, including the *bourrée*, *courante* and minuet. The long minuet, which opened proceedings and often went on for a considerable time, was more of an introduction than a dance. It was presided over by Nash who, in strict order of social precedence, introduced each man present to a partner. The couple then danced a complete figure before the lady retired and Nash introduced the man to a new partner. The second half, which followed after a lengthy supper interval, consisted of country dances. The dress code for dances was extremely formal with gentlemen required to wear full wigs and ladies dresses with hoops and lappets hanging from their shoulders. Dancing finished at 11 p.m. prompt to allow members of the Company to return to their lodgings and rest in preparation for the following morning's early start at the baths. Sunday evenings offered a variety of church services and sacred oratorios.

Commenting on Beau Nash's achievements in the biography he wrote in 1762, Oliver Goldsmith gushed: 'Bath yields a continuous rotation of diversions, and people of all ways of thinking, even from the libertine to the Methodist, have it in their power to complete the day with employments suited to their inclinations' (Goldsmith 1762: 48). Several distinguished visitors from abroad echoed this positive verdict and were struck by the spa's elegance and refinement. During a stay in 1794, Joseph Haydn declared it 'one of the most beautiful cities in Europe'. By comparison, Continental spas often seemed very dull. A *curiste* in Vichy in the later eighteenth century reported that 'one goes at six in the morning to the fountain and finds that everyone is already there. One drinks, then walks around the fountain, then takes a long promenade, and then drinks more of the disagreeable water. This is what one does until midday.' She went on to note that the afternoon and evening were no more fun with none of the diversions and distractions provided at Bath (Mackaman 1998: 18). The main nocturnal excitement in Aix-les-Bains was the reported appearance of a vicious breed of snakes in the baths.

Some of Bath's more regular English visitors were rather less enamoured of its charms, which they felt were only surface-deep. The composer Charles Dibdin noted in 1787, 'at Bath everything is superficial' (Dibdin 1788: 35). He complained that Bath audiences greeted all musical performances, which attracted leading soloists and players from across Europe, with 'a vacant gravity, an unfeeling stare, a milk and water indifference' and added 'Heaven defend me from such a set of insipid, vague, unmeaning countenances' (Dibdin 1788: 24). Charles Wesley, the earnest evangelical and co-founder of Methodism with his brother, John, retired to Bath in 1761 following a breakdown in his health but found it 'hell on earth' and moved back to London.

Several writers identified a hidden side to Bath in its heyday that was very much at odds with the positive spin provided by the spa doctors and promoters. An anonymous visitor around 1720 dismissed it as:

A scruffy minor spa of squalid lodgings, roving ruffians and pickpockets, quack doctors and nude bathing in unhygienic baths by visitors whose principal employments were yawning and drinking those waters which nothing but the most extraordinary fear of death could ever have reconciled any human being to touching after the first drop. (Rotherham 2014: 19–20)

Others were struck by the filth and stench. For Daniel Defoe, Bath was 'more like a prison than a place of diversion' and 'scarce gives the Company room to converse out of the smell of their own excrements' (Defoe 1928, 2: 168). Noting that it stank 'like a common sewer', he compared its low-lying location and close air unfavourably with the purer and more bracing atmosphere of Buxton. Another visitor to Bath, who simply styled himself 'a gentleman', complained in 1722 that 'the smoke and the slime of the waters, the promiscuous multitude of the people in the bath, with nothing but their heads above water, with the height of walls that environ the bath, gave me a lively idea of the several pictures I had seen of Fra Angelico's in Italy of Purgatory' (Defoe 1888: 248).

Perhaps the most graphic account of this seedy shadow side of Bath, and especially of the impurity and dirtiness of its waters, comes in Tobias Smollett's novel *The Expedition of Humphry Clinker*, published in 1771. Smollett himself suffered badly from gout, asthma and lung disease and obsessed about the state of his health. He practised for two years as a physician in Bath, not enjoying the experience very much and adopting a brusque tone with the many valetudinarians who consulted him – he told one lady that 'if she had time to play at being ill, he had not time to play at curing her.' He wrote a treatise on the external use of the mineral waters that expressed considerable doubts as to their cleanliness. He put these concerns into his account of the experiences of Matthew Bramble, the novel's hero, an elderly gout-ridden gentleman. Misanthropic, irritable, melancholic and leading a sedentary and unhealthy life, he embarks on a tour of the spas of England searching for a cure for his many illnesses.

Arriving in Bath, he finds it does nothing for the 'irritable nerves of an invalid':

> This place, which Nature and Providence seem to have intended as a resource from distemper and disquiet, is become the very centre of racket and dissipation. Instead of that peace, tranquillity and ease, so necessary to those who labour under bad health, weak nerves, and irregular spirits; here we have nothing but noise, tumult, and hurry; with the fatigue and slavery of maintaining a ceremonial, more stiff, formal, and oppressive, than the etiquette of the German elector. A National Hospital it may be; but one would imagine that none but lunatics are admitted. (Smollett 1990: 34)

The superficial aspects of Bath have a certain appeal to Bramble. He reports 'all is gaiety, good humour, and diversion. The eye is continually entertained with the splendour of dress and equipage; and the ear with the sound of coaches, chaises, chairs and other carriages. *The merry bells ring round* from morn till night' (Smollett 1990: 38). But on closer inspection the Company is not so appealing, including as it does 'the very dregs of the people' and 'every upstart of fortune':

> Agents, commissaries, and contractors, who have fattened in two successive wars on the blood of the nation; usurers, brokers, and jobbers of every kind; men of low birth, and no breeding, have found themselves suddenly translated into a state of affluence, unknown to former ages ... Knowing no other criterion of greatness, but the ostentation of wealth, they discharge their affluence without taste or conduct, through every channel of the most absurd extravagance; and all of them hurry to Bath, because here, without any further qualification, they can mingle with the princes and nobles of the land. Even the wives and

daughters of low tradesmen, who like shovel-nosed sharks, prey upon the blubber of those uncouth whales of fortune, are infected with the same rage of displaying their importance; and the slightest indisposition serves them for a pretext to insist upon being conveyed to Bath, where they may hobble country-dances and cotillions among lordlings, squires, counsellors and clergy. (Smollett 1990: 36–7)

The mixing of these nouveau riche parvenus with those of more established social status serves for Bramble to 'heighten the humour in the farce of life':

Yesterday morning, at the Pump-room, I saw a broken-winded Wapping landlady squeeze through a circle of peers, to salute her brandy-merchant, who stood by the window, prop'd upon crutches; and the paralytic attorney of Shoe-lane, in shuffling up to the bar, kicked the shins of the chancellor of England, while his lordship, in a cut bob, drank a glass of water at the pump. (Smollett 1990: 47–8)

Bramble is initially taken with the cheerfulness of the sick which 'seemed to triumph over their constitutions'. But although they seem on first acquaintance to joke about their own calamities,

I afterwards found out that they were not without their moments, and even hours of disquiet. Each of them apart, in succeeding conferences, expatiated on his own particular grievances; and they were all malcontents at bottom ... They have long left off using the waters, after having experienced their inefficacy. The diversions of the place they are not in a condition to enjoy ... In the forenoon they crawl out to the rooms or the coffee-house, where they take a hand at whist, and their evenings they murder in private parties, among peevish invalids and insipid old women. (Smollett 1990: 55)

What really repels Bramble, and here he reflected Smollett's own view, is the appalling lack of hygiene in the baths and the drinking fountains around the town.

> Two days ago I went into the King's Bath in order to clear the strainer of the skin for the benefit of a free perspiration; and the first object that saluted my eye was a child full of scrophulous ulcers, carried in the arms of one of the guides, under the very noses of the bathers. I was so shocked at the sight that I retired immediately with indignation and disgust. Suppose the matter of those ulcers, floating on the water, comes in contact with my skin when the pores are all open, I would ask you what must be the consequence? Good Heaven, the very thought makes my blood run cold! We know not what sores may be running into the waters while we are bathing and what sort of matter we may thus imbibe; the king's-evil, the scurvy, the cancer and the pox; and, no doubt, the heat will render the virus the more volatile and penetrating. (Smollett 1990: 44)

Seeking to purify himself from such contamination, Bramble turns to the more exclusive surroundings of the Duke of Kingston's private bath, only to be 'almost suffocated for want of free air, the place was so small and the steam so stifling'. Drinking the water proves equally hazardous 'for, after a long conversation with the doctor, about the construction of the pump and the cistern, it is very far from being clear with me, that the patients in the Pump-room don't swallow the scourings of the bathers.' Regurgitation from the bath into the cistern of the pump leads him to reflect 'What a delicate beveridge is every day quaffed by the drinkers, medicated with the sweat and dirt, and dandriff; and the abominable discharges of various kinds, from twenty different diseased bodies, parboiling in the kettle below.' Trying what he thinks may be a purer source, the spring supplying the private baths on the abbey green, he detects a strange taste and smell and discovers on enquiry 'that the Roman baths in this quarter were found covered by an old burying ground, belonging to the Abbey; thro' which, in all probability, the water drains in its passage: so that as we drink the decoction of living bodies at the Pump-room, we swallow the strainings of rotten bones and carcasses at the private bath' (Smollett 1990: 45).

There were other causes of contamination of Bath's thermal mineral waters. In his 1742 description of the town, John Wood commented that cats, dogs and even pigs were regularly hurled over the side of the King's Bath to the amusement of onlookers and the annoyance of bathers. There are accounts of over-enthusiastic imbibing of the waters apparently causing death. At a breakfast concert in the Assembly Room in 1741 one of the players, Ralph Thicknesse, described by his brother, Philip, as 'reckoned the best gentleman player on the fiddle in England', collapsed and died while playing first violin in one of his own concertos. The doctor who attended him gave the cause of death as a stroke brought on by anxiety over the performance of his work, but his brother reckoned that he died of 'the Bath waters' of which he had drunk plentifully earlier in the morning before eating a hearty breakfast of spongy rolls. Bathing in the waters could also prove fatal, as it seems to have been for Henry Fielding's wife, who caught a fever and died in his arms during a cure they both took in 1744. This experience did not stop Fielding himself returning to Bath to try to cure his gout nine years later. It was not just at Bath that consuming the waters could prove fatal, if an epitaph in a Cheltenham graveyard is to be believed:

Here lies I and my three daughters,
Kill'd by drinking Cheltenham waters;
If we had stuck to Epsom salts,
We'd not been a lying in these here vaults.

Alongside the lack of hygiene in the list of Bath's hidden *Kurschatten* went its reputation for sexual improprieties and amorous liaisons. The 'panting breasts' and 'vigorous sparks' that Ned Ward had observed at the baths in the 1690s (see page 91) did not disappear with the stricter and outwardly decorous regime introduced by Nash.The Company chose to emulate his example rather than follow his moralistic rules, as an anonymous piece of doggerel dating from the 1720s confirms:

> There is a place down in a gloomy vale,
> Where burthen'd Nature lays her nasty tail;
> Ten thousand pilgrims thither do resort
> For ease, disease, for lechery and sport.
> Here Lords and Ladies, and the Devil and all,
> Resort in clusters, at the Spring and Fall;
> Here beauteous females in conception flow
> By genial Waters, soon more fertile grow,
> Here barren ladies may their wants relieve
> But by the waters only they conceive.

The idea that bathing in the thermal waters stimulated conception among the barren undoubtedly attracted many women to Bath. If they returned home fertile, it was likely to be because of the attentions of gentlemen bathers rather than anything in the water. There are numerous accounts of couplings and sexual shenanigans taking place in the baths. Thomas D'Urfey's comedy *The Bath: Or, The Western Lass*, published in 1701, opens with the observation that it was not uncommon for a voluptuous lady to plunge naked into the waters, 'and if there be e'r a plump Londoner there … he's on the back of her in a trice, and tabering her Buttocks round the Bath as if he were beating a Drum' (D'Urfey 1701: 1). Daniel Defoe noted on his 1720 visit that while 'the ladies and the gentlemen pretend to keep some distance, and each to their proper side', they 'mingle' nonetheless, 'and talk, rally, make vows, and sometimes love' (Defoe 1928, 2: 34). In 1737, Bath Corporation felt the need to make an order 'that no Male Person above the age of Ten years shall at any time hereafter go into any Bath or Baths within this City by day or by night without a Pair of Drawers and a Waistcoat on their bodies' and 'that no Female Person shall ... go into any Bath ... without a decent Shift on their bodies' (Fawcett 1995: 90). But amatory adventures among the bathers continued as Anstey's *New Bath Guide* enthusiastically confirms:

> 'Twas a glorious sight to behold the fair sex
> All wading with gentlemen up to their necks,
> And view them so prettily tumble and sprawl
> In a great soaking kettle as big as a hall. (Anstey 1770: 38)

The association of bath houses with brothels that had begun in the Middle Ages persisted through the eighteenth century. The word 'bagnio' came into general use throughout Britain from the 1720s onwards to signify a brothel, with the working girls being known as 'nymphs'. There was a particular concentration of such places in and around Covent Garden and Drury Lane in London, marking the beginning of the Soho sex industry, and there were also many bagnios in Bath. Several prominent novels and plays from the period confirm the spa's reputation for amatory adventures and illicit liaisons. The eponymous heroine of Daniel Defoe's *Moll Flanders* (1722) reflects that Bath is a place 'where men find a mistress sometimes, but very rarely look for a wife'. Henry Fielding's *Tom Jones* (1749) provides racy accounts of cavorting in the baths and flirting in the Assembly and Pump rooms. Richard Sheridan's 1777 play, *The School for Scandal*, describes the goings-on in Bath, which the author observed during his residence there. It was not just the baths that offered opportunities for flirting. At a concert in the New Rooms in April 1778 the radical politician, John Wilkes, was 'seen to be paying more attention to the fire in Mrs Stafford's eyes than to the silvery voice of Miss Cantelo or to the graceful rendering of selections from the *Messiah*' (Bradley 2010: 43). Henry Fielding enjoyed eyeing up beautiful girls in the Pump Room during his stays in Bath in the early 1740s when he took the waters in an effort to cure his gout, although he complained that there was a general lack of attractive women and that the spa was 'full of nothing but noise, impertinence and confusion' (Battestin 1989: 312).

Jean-Bernard, abbé Le Blanc, a French art critic, who visited Bath in 1738, was fascinated by the transformation that young women went through during their time there: 'they are totally different here from what they are like in London and what produces this remarkable difference is the casting off of the constraint and melancholy imposed upon them by the yoke of habit in the Capital, for one month of liberty and diversion' (Le Blanc 1751: 333). Somewhat surprisingly, given all the opportunities that the spa seemed to offer men to take advantage of women, Le Blanc regarded Bath as a female-friendly environment. He believed that its atmosphere was especially liberating for women, for whom a cure there was '*un séjour d'enchantement*' (a stay of enchantment). It is certainly true that some of the ladies who took the waters there were rather more enthusiastic about the experience than many of the men who wrote about it. One such was Hester Piozzi, the diarist and author who was a close friend of Dr Johnson. She spent the 1791 season in Bath, persuaded by her Italian husband that the waters would cure her stomach pains and also 'carry away his little nervous complaints' and found her stay hugely restorative: 'Here I have good Air and good Water and good Company – and at last– *good Nights* so that I mean to be among the merriest immediately' (Dolan 2001: 147).

It is striking how many English ladies visited Continental spas. Brian Dolan points out in his book *Ladies of the Grand Tour* that 'travelling abroad for the sake of one's health was one of the few legitimate reasons women in Enlightenment England could use to escape domestic circumstances. Such was the attraction of these liberties that many sought shelter in the temple of health who did not require Hygeia's services' (Dolan 2001: 160). For their aristocratic female patrons, the appeal of Continental spas lay as much in their cosmopolitan social diversity as in the benefits of their waters and the pleasures of their diversions. As Lady Elizabeth

Montagu commented during a visit to Spa in 1763, 'here you meet all the various orders and professions in which mankind are classed' (Dolan 2001: 148). Spa seems to have been a particular favourite of these pioneer female tourists, although a stay there could bring embarrassing moments. Jean-Philippe de Limbourg, one of Spa's leading physicians, wrote with some amusement in 1764 about a journey back into town by a group of *curistes* who had ventured out to drink copiously from the renowned but rather remote *source de la Géronstère*. It was, he noted, 'attended by some little inconveniences, or embarrassments, especially to the ladies' who were obliged to stop frequently en route so that 'one, perhaps, finds out a commodious place behind some large stone, and another screens herself behind a bush' (de Limbourg 1764: 71–2).

A visit by Peter the Great in 1717 helped to establish Spa as one of the most fashionable Continental watering places. He managed to cure his liver and digestive problems by drinking up to twenty-one glasses from the *source de la Géronstère* every morning for a month. He travelled out to the source in a chaise drawn by two horses but usually walked back – needing, I would imagine, as I did when I returned from drinking several glasses there, to relieve himself several times on the way. He recorded his thanks for the cure in a Latin inscription on a marble tablet that can still be seen beside the town's most central drinking fountain, which is named after him, the *source du Pouhon Pierre-le-Grand*. In 1734, Baron Karl Ludwig von Pöllnitz, chamberlain to the Prussian Court, wrote a guidebook entitled *Amusemens des eaux de Spa*. Translated into English and German two years later, it was the first guidebook to a spa that focused on the diversions and amusements available to visitors rather than on the chemical composition and therapeutic benefits of the water. It spawned a host of imitators, with similar guides being published in English, German and French to Bad Schwalbach and Wiesbaden in 1738, Baden bei Zürich and Pfäfers in 1739 and Baden bei Wien in 1747. They played a key role in promoting these spas as pleasure resorts for those in good health seeking distraction and not just as cure centres for invalids. Spa led the way in other respects, publishing from 1751 a weekly list of guests with their titles and nationalities. This practice, which continued until 1939, was widely taken up by other spas, enhancing their social cachet by appealing to the vanity and snobbery of their clientele.

Spa's hedonistic attractions were much enhanced by the opening of a casino, known as La Redoute, in 1763. It is the second-oldest casino in Europe, with only one built in Venice in 1638 pre-dating it. A theatre was added in 1769, and the following year a ballroom and second gaming room were provided in a building situated in a landscaped park and named Le Waux-Hall after Vauxhall in London, famous for its pleasure gardens. A third casino, Salon Levez, opened in Spa in 1785. Rivalry between the three establishments became so heated that it escalated into violence and the prince-bishop of Liège, who owned La Redoute and benefited from its revenues, had to send in 200 men and two cannons to restore order. Regulations were subsequently drawn up to divide concerts, balls and assemblies equitably between the three establishments. Spa now had all the essential accoutrements of a fashionable *ville d'eau* and attracted aristocratic patrons from across Europe. More than 140 mansions were built in the town between 1740 and 1780 and one visitor in the 1770s counted thirty titled princes in the list of *curistes*. The aristocratic visitors were dubbed '*bobelins*' by the locals – there is some uncertainty as to whether this phrase was derived from the Latin word '*bibelus*', meaning a great drinker, or from a Walloon expression denoting weird and eccentric behaviour. It is clear from the accounts of those who came for the season that it was the distractions rather than the waters that proved Spa's main attraction. Staying there for the summer months of 1768, the Earl of Carlisle reported to a friend: 'I rise at six; am on horseback at breakfast; play at cricket till dinner; and dance in the evening till I can scarce crawl to bed at eleven. This is a life for you.' (Hibbert 1969: 219)

Perhaps the most famous visitor to Spa in this period was Giacomo Casanova, the Italian adventurer who has gone down in history as the world's most notorious womaniser. During a stay in 1772, he described it as 'the enclosure where all the nations of Europe come once a year, in the summer, to make a thousand follies'. He attempted to have his evil way with a young girl called Mercy but when he put his hand under the bedclothes to seduce her, she responded by punching him so hard on the nose that the blood ran and he saw stars, which 'quite extinguished the fire of my concupiscence'. It was, in fact, gambling rather than love-making that he saw as the main concern of his fellow *curistes*:

> The number of adventurers who flock to Spa during the season is something incredible, and they all hope to make their fortunes; and, as may be supposed, most of them go away as naked as they came, if not more so. Money circulates with great freedom, but principally amongst the gamesters, shop-keepers, money-lenders, and courtezans. The money which proceeds from the gaming-table has three issues: the first and smallest share goes to the Prince-Bishop of Liège; the second and larger portion, to the numerous amateur cheats who frequent the place; and by far the largest of all to the coffers of twelve sharpers, who keep the tables and are authorised by the sovereign.
>
> Thus goes the money. It comes from the pockets of the dupes – poor moths who burn their wings at Spa!
>
> The Wells are a mere pretext for gaming, intriguing, and fortune-hunting. There are a few honest people who go for amusement, and a few for rest and relaxation after the toils of business. (de Seingalt 1894: 28)

Rather disappointingly, Casanova has been airbrushed out of Spa's official historical record. He does not appear on the huge wall painting dating from 1894 and known as the *Livre d'Or*, which shows ninety-one famous visitors to the town and is now on display in the Tourist Office.

Spa's cosmopolitan atmosphere was confirmed in 1781 when it received the title of 'the café of Europe'. This appellation is usually credited to the Habsburg Emperor Joseph II, who visited Spa that year, though the phrase also appeared in a book of poems and songs that possibly pre-dated his visit. Imperial patronage similarly benefited Baden bei Wien. Emperor Joseph I first came for treatment at the Frauenbad there in 1707 and returned on several occasions. Even more important were the later visits of the Empress Maria Theresa, who gave her name to one of the main bath houses and to the *Kurpark* gardens.

Baden bei Wien's most famous guest in the eighteenth century, Wolfgang Mozart, did not come to take the waters himself but rather to visit his sick wife, Constanze. Between 1783 and 1791 she gave birth to six children, only two of whom survived beyond infancy. The strain of almost constant pregnancy, and complications surrounding most of the births, put her into a state of chronic ill health. A series of lengthy treatments at Baden was prescribed and between 1789 and 1791 she spent several weeks at a time there, often accompanied by her young son, Karl, and her husband's pupil, Franz Süssmayr. Mozart wrote to friends and patrons imploring them to help with the considerable costs of the cures, telling one 'she will have to take the baths sixty times – and later on in the year she will have to go out there again. God grant that it may do her good' (Bradley 2010: 61). Although he remained at home in Vienna working, he wrote to Constanze almost daily, sending her gifts to aid her recovery, including infusions, electuaries and ants' eggs, and visited her regularly.

Although there is no evidence that Mozart himself ever tried bathing in the Baden waters to ease the rheumatic fever from which he suffered in his latter years, he seems to have been an enthusiast for spa treatments, despite their heavy cost. Writing to Constanze from Munich in November 1790, he suggested that the two of them should make a journey further afield to some German spas 'so that you may try some other waters'. It was, however, to Baden bei Wien that she returned the following June, now pregnant with their sixth child. Mozart, who was in the middle of composing *Die Zauberflöte* (*The Magic Flute*), wrote to her advising 'When you are bathing, do take care not to slip and never stay in alone. If I were you I should occasionally omit a day in order not to do the cure too violently' (Bradley 2010: 61). Constanze seems not to have heeded his subsequent advice that she should 'take the baths only every other day, and then only for an hour' and in response to a report that she had a stomach upset, he found himself asking 'Perhaps the baths are having a too laxative effect? My advice is that you should stop them now! Today is the day when you are not supposed to take one and yet I wager that that little wife of mine has been to the baths. Seriously I had much rather you would prolong your cure well into the autumn' (Bradley 2010: 62–3).

When Constanze eventually returned home from her last cure in mid-October 1791, she found her husband exhausted from overwork. In her absence, he had regularly risen at 4.30 a.m. and worked on until midnight, completing his Clarinet Concerto and his Requiem. He became progressively weaker and died on 5 December, just three weeks short of his thirty-sixth birthday. Mozart's biographers have speculated whether he packed Constanze off to Baden to be rid of her so that he could pursue amatory affairs in Vienna as well as getting on with his work. They have also wondered whether she had an affair with Süssmayr while there and why her husband sent his young assistant off with her rather than keeping him in Vienna to help him. It is difficult to make a judgement on these questions. Perhaps the more intriguing question is whether Mozart would have survived longer if he had himself taken a cure for his rheumatic fever.

Baden bei Zürich was also gaining popularity at this time, although it lacked the imperial patronage of its Austrian namesake. It too had its shadow side behind a glittering and elegant façade. David-François de Merveilleux, who came to take a cure there in 1738, found the place dirty and decadent, with women and men bathing together naked, the water tasting of rotten eggs or urine, and the glamour of the balls rather marred by the appearance of the young ladies: 'After they have danced a lot and are consequently sweating a good deal, lice emerge from their beautiful hair, causing some distress.' It was the German women who were most infested — their habit of applying huge quantities of powder without combing their hair properly made 'it not surprising that these animals, who like delicate flesh, multiply so much'. There was just one redeeming feature about this unpleasant state of affairs: 'These girls have such beautiful skin that it is a pleasure to remove these vermin as soon as they appear' (Mercier 1922: 69). The other leading Swiss spa, Pfäfers, was meanwhile being literally brought out of the shadows and given a more salubrious and appealing atmosphere. Between 1704 and 1718 the abbot of the Benedictine monastery, which continued to own and administer the baths, built an elegant new baroque bath house at the entrance to the Tamina Gorge, to which thermal water was piped from the spring deep inside it. This meant that those taking a cure there no longer had to make the perilous descent down the cliffs. The bath house was extended to provide accommodation for up to 500 guests. Finally closed in 1969, it now houses a museum devoted to the history of the old Bad Pfäfers, complete with surviving baths, a restaurant and concert hall.

The Bohemian spa of Karlsbad, with its eighty-one thermal mineral springs, was also on the rise. Like Spa, it benefited from the patronage of Peter the Great, who took cures there in 1711 and 1712, and became known as Adelsbad, or the spa of the nobility, because of its aristocratic clientele. Johann Goethe made the first of his many visits there in 1785, telling a friend that the experience of taking a cure had plunged him into 'a laziness beyond all description' and that he needed 'to find a little sexual adventure' if he was not to die of boredom during his forty-five-day stay. While taking a cure there in 1795, ostensibly to cure a bout of tonsillitis, he fell in love with a poetess, Friederike Brun, with whom he walked up and down in the pump room drinking sulphurous waters. He rose at 5 a.m. every morning just so that he could be sure of accompanying her. Overall, Goethe made thirteen visits to Karlsbad, often staying for several months at a time. There is a white marble bust of him beside the path bearing his name that runs alongside the River Teplá from the Grandhotel Pupp to the art gallery. Engraved on a plaque next to it is a verse in which he noted that a list of all the joys, realisations and sensations that he had experienced there would take far too long to confess.

Overall, during the eighteenth century the regime required of spa patients was made much more precise and reduced in its severity. In Karlsbad at the beginning of the century it was common for people to be drinking seventy or more cups of thermal water (around nine to ten litres) a day. This induced severe diarrhoea, which was regarded as an important if unpleasant part of the therapy, having the effect of removing internal parasites and cleaning out the system. Dr David Becher, who started practising in Karlsbad in 1758 and wrote several treatises about its waters, was influential in changing the nature of the cure there. Seeing no therapeutic advantages in inducing diarrhoea through excessive intake of the waters, nor in bathing in them for long hours, he cut down the requirements to just a few glasses of water in the morning and evening and no more than an hour in the baths. His much more palatable regime, involving a pyramid cure where the amount of water taken was gradually increased, reaching a peak in the middle week of the typical three-week stay and then tailing off towards the end, was widely taken up in other Continental spas. Among Becher's patients was Friedrich Schiller, to whom Goethe had recommended a cure in Karlsbad on the grounds that 'one could travel a hundred miles and not see so many interesting people.' He sought treatment for his pneumonia there in 1791, drinking eighteen cups a day of its sodium-rich waters. His one and only visit there is commemorated in a rather stark art nouveau monument erected in 1909 near the town art gallery.

The Continental spas, which really came into their own in the nineteenth century, will dominate the next three chapters. To conclude this one it is appropriate to return to England at the very end of the eighteenth century and to note two spa romances among prominent members of the staunchly evangelical Clapham Sect, which played a key role in cleaning up English society and paved the way for Victorian propriety and seriousness. The first took place in 1790 in Buxton, which had just received a considerable boost with the erection of the elegant Crescent by the fifth Duke of Devonshire, where Marianne Sykes was taking the waters in an effort to alleviate mild depression. She told her mother 'This horrid water disagreed with me' and that she was shunning the frivolities of spa society in favour of solitary rambles 'over these bleak moors in quest of misery', seeking out the homes of very poor people and playing the lady bountiful – 'a few shillings gratifies them and I leave them I hope not unimproved by the acquaintance' (Stott 2012: 41). Alongside this high-minded charitable activity, she found time to indulge in a more traditional spa pastime, hanging out with the handsome evangelical banker Henry Thornton, who probed the state of her soul and lectured her 'on the duty of preserving my health'. Knowing that her mother would not approve of too much intimacy, Marianne assured her that she had only admitted him to her party once, and 'then I could not well decline it, for he had dined with us – it was Sunday and we were the only Spa people at Church in the afternoon, and as he earnestly requested it I thought I might as well let him come with me as walk home with him to the Crescent in full view of everybody' (Stott 2012: 42). Henry and Marianne proceeded very circumspectly with their relationship, which eventually led to marriage. He promised to remain in Buxton until her doctor confirmed that she was in good health, meanwhile securing her full conversion to the 'vital religion' of evangelicalism.

Marianne's close friend, William Wilberforce, the best-known figure in the Clapham Sect, had something much closer to a classic *Kurschatten* experience while undertaking spa cures. He had joined her in Buxton, and indeed she had fallen a little in love with him there before turning her attention to Henry Thornton. In 1796, returning there for the summer months, he became smitten with a young lady taking the waters, Miss Dawes, but concluded that at eighteen she was too young for him – he was thirty-seven. This episode, coupled with the news that another old flame was getting married, threw him into a state of turmoil and agonising as to whether he would ever find the right companion. The following year, he spent Easter at Bath and took tea with a Miss Spooner. He found her very attractive but was too shy to talk to her. On Easter Sunday he went to the fashionable Laura Chapel and found his mind 'sadly rambling' throughout the sermon with thoughts of her. He felt that he was 'in danger of falling in Love with [a] Creature of my own Imagination' (Stott 2012: 73). This classic *Kurschatten* in fact turned into a solid and lasting relationship. Wilberforce and Barbara Spooner went together to the Pump Room on a number of occasions. A week after their first meeting he took supper with her family and declared himself 'captivated' by her. The courtship proceeded in a suitably proper and seemly manner and they married the following year.

In 1790 Horace Walpole, the essayist and Whig politician who strongly supported Wilberforce in his crusade to abolish the slave trade, observed: 'One would think the English were ducks: they are forever waddling to the waters.' It was, however, to the seaside rather than to the inland spas that his compatriots were increasingly waddling to satisfy their aquatic cravings. Sea bathing was being widely canvassed as a healthier and more hygienic alternative to immersion in scum-clad mineral water baths. As early as 1750, Richard Russell, a physician based in Lewes, Sussex, published a dissertation recommending the use of seawater to treat glandular diseases. It was the first major work to argue the case for the therapeutic benefits of drinking and bathing in seawater. Russell became a national celebrity and moved his medical practice to Brighton, which came to eclipse Bath as the nation's premiere resort, thanks in large part to the decision of the Prince Regent, later George IV, to take his patronage and his mistresses there. He first went to Brighton in 1783 and returned annually for the next forty years. His father, George III, who similarly preferred bathing in the sea to inland spas, favoured Weymouth, which he first visited in 1789. Many of their subjects followed this royal example with several, like Susannah Wedgwood, hedging their bets by combining both forms of therapy – in an effort to cure her rheumatism she took the waters at both Bath and Bristol Hotwells in the spring of 1791 and then spent the summer bathing at Weymouth. Tobias Smollett was a notable advocate of sea bathing, having taken it up to ease his own lung complaints in the 1760s. Significantly, he had Matthew Bramble declare in *The Expedition of Humphry Clinker* that, after failing to find any relief from his gout at either Bath or Harrogate, he was resolved to make his way to Scarborough 'where I propose to brace up my fibres by sea-bathing' (Smollett 1990: 168). A growing number of doctors were coming to the view that the sea rather than the spa was where health-giving benefits were to be gained. William Heberden, a leading London physician, noted shortly before his death in 1801: 'I have not been able to observe any good in arthritic cases from the external use of these [Bath]waters ... Sea-bathing has contributed far more to recover the strength of gouty persons' (Porter and Rousseau 1998: 126).

Where their Georgian predecessors had gone to inland spas for their health and entertainment, the Victorians went to the seaside. A new and even more popular kind of resort emerged with bathing machines on the beach, a long pier stretching out into the sea, promenades, donkey rides and Pierrot shows. It was perhaps not surprising that the British with their maritime heritage and traditions should take to the sea in such a big way around the time of Nelson and Trafalgar. It has been argued that the British love of the seaside might indeed have spread to the Continent were it not for the sudden stop that the Napoleonic Wars put to the Grand Tours by English aristocrats. As it was, thalassotherapy (the use of seawater for therapeutic purposes) did develop in France and Italy, and is still practised there, but Continental Europeans as a whole, especially in the landlocked countries of Central and Eastern Europe, stuck to their thermal mineral springs and spas.

There were other reasons for the decline of the British spas at the end of the eighteenth century. The Napoleonic Wars deprived them of men and left their female guests pining and bereft – as one reported from Buxton in 1798: 'the male youth and middle life of England are all soldiered and gone to camps and coasts, and so a few prim parsons and a few dancing doctors are the forlorn hope of the belles' (Langham and Wells 2005: 39). Several of those who might have been expected to frequent spas started taking to drugs as an alternative way of dealing with their hypochondria and chronic sickness. Samuel Taylor Coleridge was a prime example. Suffering rheumatic fever, gout and neuralgia as a young man in the late 1790s, he started to consume large quantities of opiates on a regular basis, a practice that he continued for the rest of his life. There were high levels of addiction to opium in Victorian Britain, not least among the upper and literary classes. For hypochondriacs and those suffering from nervous conditions, which would now probably be categorised as depression or schizophrenia, it provided the relief and escape that an earlier generation had sought through a spa cure. One of those who joined Coleridge in his opium binges was Tom Wedgwood, who had been prescribed spa cures by two leading doctors for his hypochondria (see page 38). He died at the age of thirty-four in 1805 as a direct result of his addiction to opium and other drugs. Sometimes both approaches were combined, as in the case of Helen Gladstone (see page 23). In a rather healthier development, scientific progress made it possible for people to enjoy the taste and benefits of mineral water without the need to visit a spa. Johann Jacob Schweppe, a German-Swiss watchmaker and amateur scientist, developed the first practical process to manufacture bottled carbonated mineral water. He founded the Schweppes Company in Geneva in 1783 and moved to London in 1792. Schweppes mineral and tonic water, with its supposed therapeutic benefits, became extremely popular, thanks in part to its enthusiastic endorsement by Erasmus Darwin and to its adoption by William IV in 1831, giving the company a royal warrant.

Although the Regency period marked the end of the heyday of England's spas and of Bath in particular, some other English watering places actually grew in popularity in the early nineteenth century, notably Leamington and Cheltenham. However, they continued to have a rather dubious reputation, which was played up by writers and journalists. William Cobbett, who was something of a professional taker of a low view, had some typically trenchant comments on the hidden shadow side of spas in general, and Cheltenham in particular, in his *Rural Rides* of 1826:

> Cheltenham is what they call a 'watering place'; that is to say, a place to which East India plunderers, West India floggers, English tax-gorgers, together with gluttons, drunkards, and debauchees of all descriptions, female as well as male, resort, at the suggestion of silently laughing quacks, in the hope of getting rid of the bodily consequences of their manifold sins and iniquities. When I enter a place like this, I always feel disposed to squeeze up my nose with my fingers. It is nonsense, to be sure; but I conceit that every two-legged creature that I see coming near me is about to cover me with the poisonous proceeds of its impurities. To places like this come all that is knavish and all that is foolish and all that is base; gamesters, pickpockets, and harlots; young wife-hunters in search of rich and ugly and old women, and young husband-hunters in search of rich and wrinkled or half-rotten men ... It is situated in a nasty, flat, stupid spot, without anything pleasant near it. (Cobbett 1934: 411)

English watering places will feature little in the rest of this book, being almost wholly eclipsed throughout the nineteenth and twentieth centuries by Continental spas. Before we leave them let us take a last look at Bath, the model and prototype for the modern European spa, through the eyes of two perceptive observers who caught its ambiguity and hidden shadow side at the end of its golden age. The first, Benjamin Silliman, an earnest young American scientist, found that a visit there in 1805 left him with mixed emotions. At one level, he found it 'the most beautiful city in England ... and the most magnificent in the structure of its buildings'. Yet he went on to add: 'It is probably the most dissipated place in the kingdom. It is resorted to by many real invalids but by far the greater number belong to that class who wear away life in a round of fashionable frivolities, without moral aim or intellectual dignity' (Silliman 1810: 22, 23, 24).

A more nuanced picture of Bath, which perhaps even more clearly emphasises its shadow side, emerges from the novels of Jane Austen, three of which were partially set in the spa town. She and her sister were reluctantly dragged to live in Bath in 1801 by their father and mother, largely because of the latter's hypochondria. Jane described her first impression of the city, as seen from Kingsdown Hill, as 'all vapour, shadow, smoke and confusion' (Chapman 1952: 123). If this phrase emphasised physical and climatic features, it also hinted at a deeper, almost spiritual malaise. She found living there enervating and stifling and she pined to get back to the wholesomeness and simplicity of Steventon, the Hampshire village where she had grown up. She also found living in Bath very lonely, an aspect conveyed in her novel *Northanger Abbey*, where she has Mrs Allen reflect more than once 'What a delightful place Bath is, and how pleasant it would be if we had any acquaintances here' (Austen 1960: 27), a statement that underlines the sense of isolation existing in the midst of the shallow bonhomie of the Company. Another novel, *Emma*, further highlights the frustration and superficiality of spa life. Its central male characters are Mr Henry Woodhouse, a hypochondriac who tries the waters in Bath several times unsuccessfully in an attempt to ease his many ailments, and the Rev. Philip Elton, a social-climbing clergyman who takes refuge there after being spurned by Emma and returns after a few weeks with the pretentious, nouveau riche Jane who becomes his wife.

Jane Austen found the atmosphere of Bath unconducive to her muse and wrote almost nothing during the four years that she lived there. She put much of her frustration into the character of Anne Elliot, the heroine of her last complete novel, *Persuasion*, who feels

stifled and trapped in the dull, formal, artificial atmosphere of
the spa town, with its company of 'sauntering politicians, bustling
housekeepers and flirting girls' and longs to return to the more
bracing air of the Dorset seaside resort of Lyme Regis. Significantly,
the novel on which Austen was working at the time of her death in
1817, *Sanditon*, describes the rise of a fictional seaside resort on the
south coast of England and the attempts to lure tourists there by
building assembly rooms, hotels, lodgings and shops.

Persuasion provides a powerful evocation of the largely hidden
half-life of the long-term spa resident. After visiting the Bath
lodgings of her old governess, Mrs Smith, widowed and crippled
with rheumatic fever, Anne reflects:

> She had no child to connect her with life and happiness again,
> no relations to assist in the arrangement of perplexed affairs, no
> health to make all the rest supportable. Her accommodations
> were limited to a noisy parlour, and a dark bedroom behind, with
> no possibility of moving from one to the other without assistance,
> which there was only one servant in the house to afford, and she
> never quitted the house but to be conveyed into the warm bath.
> (Austen 1961: 144)

Although Anne is struck by Mrs Smith's fortitude and capacity to
make the best of things, she cannot avoid concluding that hers is
a life simply of watching, observing and reflecting rather than of
actively doing or enjoying anything. Such was the existence lived
out by many of those who took themselves to spas and ended up
staying in them, often racked by pain or gripped by hypochondria
and obsessive introspection. For them *der Kurschatten* was not
some fleeting affair or imaginary romance but rather a shadow of
permanent melancholic loneliness.

5

THE NINETEENTH CENTURY –
BADEN-BADEN BECOMES THE
BOULEVARD OF EUROPE

The nineteenth century saw the flourishing of spas across Continental Europe, notably in France, Germany and throughout the Austro-Hungarian Empire, with a growing clientele increasingly drawn from the middle classes as well as the aristocracy and a steady shift of emphasis from medical benefits to diversions and pleasures. As a song in a musical comedy from 1822 about life in the French *ville d'eau* of Le Mont-Dore enthused, 'gaiety takes the place of health'. Cures generally became less extreme and unpleasant during this period. The quantity of water prescribed for daily drinking dropped dramatically, often to just a pint or so. The length of time recommended for bathing was also shortened. Partly for reasons of hygiene and also in deference to the increasingly dominant bourgeois morality, there was more segregation of the sexes and fewer communal baths, with most guests taking their treatments in individual cabins. One spa in particular, Baden-Baden, situated in the Grand Duchy of Baden in what became the south-western corner of the German Empire, came to epitomise the cosmopolitan elegance and decadence of the European spa scene as a whole.

Some indication of the significance of spas in the cultural and social life of Europe in this period can be gleaned from the list of leading novelists who chose them as settings for their books. They include George Eliot and William Thackeray from England, Mark Twain and Henry James from the United States, George Sand, Gustave Flaubert and Alexandre Dumas from France and the Russian novelists Leo Tolstoy, Fyodor Dostoyevsky, Ivan Turgenev and Nikolai Gogol. Their novels are for the most part based on the personal experience of the authors who, like many of their contemporaries, went to spas in search of both health and hedonism. From the middle of the century especially, these spa novels focus on pleasure and diversion and hardly mention the therapeutic aspects of the waters. The *Kurschatten* theme looms large in many of them, as does an emphasis on the rich cosmopolitan atmosphere of the *Kurorte* and *villes d'eaux*. This is certainly the case in what is widely regarded as perhaps the greatest novel of the century, Tolstoy's *Anna Karenina* (1877). Much of its second part is set in the German spa of Bad Soden where Kitty Shcherbátsky is taking a successful cure for her tubercular condition. Her father, meanwhile, embarks on a tour of prominent European watering places, embracing Karlsbad, Baden-Baden and Bad Kissingen, not for any therapeutic purpose, nor even for their diversions, but rather to meet his many Russian friends who are staying in them.

In France, where the annual number of *curistes* increased from 30,000 in 1822 to over 140,000 in 1855, spas really took off during the period of the Second Empire (1852–70). By 1882, over a thousand places carried the designation *ville d'eau*, which had first appeared in the 1850s. Many were highly specialised in the treatments that they offered. According to the French historian Theodore Zeldin, Cauterets, Eaux-Bonnes and Le Mont-Dore focused on those with throat conditions and attracted numerous actors and singers, Saint-Sauveur concentrated on female neuralgia, hysteria and hypochondria, while Plombières developed a particular reputation for other gynaecological complaints, notably infertility. Emperor Napoleon III was an enthusiastic *curiste* and his visits to Vichy to treat his gout helped to establish it as the Queen of the French spas. The number of *curistes* going there rose from 575 in 1833 to around 20,000 in 1860 and over 100,000 by 1890.

German *Kurorte* enjoyed similar expansion. The number of annual *Kurgäste* at Bad Ems increased ten-fold from 652 in 1817 to 6,679 in 1857 and continued to grow even more spectacularly, reaching a peak of 12,166 in 1871. Those coming to Baden-Baden increased from 11,356 in 1832 to 70,908 in 1902. A *Bäder Lexikon* published in 1883 listed 652 *Kurorte* ranging alphabetically from Aachen to Zopport. They had a distinctive common ambience, well caught in Ellen Wood's description of the mythical German spa of Stalkenberg in her 1861 novel, *East Lynne*:

> Stalkenberg differed in no wise from the other baths of its class in the *Vaterland*. It had its linden-trees, its fair scenery, its *Kursaal*, its balls, its concerts, its gaming tables, its promenades, and its waters. The last were advertised – and some accorded their belief – to cure every malady known or imagined, from apoplexy down to an attack of love-fever, provided you only took enough of them. (Wood 2008: 385)

Within the Austro-Hungarian Empire, Bohemia came to gain a particular reputation for its spas, of which the most famous were Karlsbad and Marienbad. While the former was already well established thanks to the reputation and influence of Dr Becher and other spa physicians, the latter only developed as a spa in the 1800s. This was as the result of the combined efforts of a cleric, Karl Reitenberger, abbot of the Premonstratensian Abbey of Teplá, who was keen to exploit the mineral and gaseous waters that bubbled up through the marshy monastic lands, and a doctor, Josef Nehr, the medical officer at the monastery, who made extensive studies of the chemical composition of the waters and realised their therapeutic potential. The first bath houses and fountains were erected in 1808 and the spa was named Marienbad after the main spring, which was dedicated to the Virgin Mary. Neoclassical colonnades and pavilions were built over the main springs in the 1820s and Marienbad gradually established itself as a fashionable resort specialising in 'the reduction of corpulency and the treatment of cases of plethora and abdominal congestion in the overfed and sedentary' (Yeo 1904: 254–5).

Meanwhile, other Continental spas which had established their reputation in the eighteenth century continued to grow. The baths at Spa were rebuilt in ever grander form in 1827, 1841 and 1868 and in 1878 a *Kursaal* for concerts and exhibitions was added in the shape of a covered gallery named after King Leopold II of Belgium. Spa attracted an eclectic and eccentric clientele. The composer Giacomo Meyerbeer became well known for riding a donkey along the Avenue of Trees, while the Duchess of Orleans rode around the town on a camel. Baden bei Wien similarly built on its earlier success. Emperor Francis I stayed there with the imperial court every summer from 1803 to 1835. The first guest list, compiled in 1805, showed 2,189 *Kurgäste*; by 1878 the number had risen to 10,347. They bathed in the magnificent Römertherme, designed by the architects of the Vienna State Opera and built between 1846 and 1848. Ragaz entered the ranks of leading European spas when, following the closure of the Benedictine monastery at Pfäfers in 1838, a pipeline was constructed to bring the thermal water from the Tamina Gorge to the village. It was completed in 1840 and led to the building of several grand spa hotels, notably the Hof and later the Quellenhof, opened in 1869 by Bernhard Simon, a Swiss architect who had made his name in St Petersburg. In 1871 he designed the first indoor thermal water bathing pool in Europe, which was housed in a wooden shed adjacent to the hotel.

The spas of Central Europe benefited in the early part of the nineteenth century from the patronage of well-known writers and musicians. Among the most dedicated *Kurgäste* was Ludwig van Beethoven, who resorted to *Kurorte* in Austria and Bohemia for several months every summer in an effort to treat his multitude of medical complaints. A classic hypochondriac in both the original and the more modern meaning of the term, Beethoven was in poor health for most of his life and had a constant fear of mortal illness and an early death. The tinnitus-like condition that made him increasingly deaf was accompanied from 1801 onwards by almost permanent colitis with abdominal pain, constipation, diarrhoea and wind, compounded by persistent severe catarrh and recurrent hepatitis and jaundice. The many doctors whom he consulted, while being uncertain in their diagnosis of his actual condition, were agreed in recommending a cure involving drinking mineral water and taking thermal baths. He made at least fourteen visits to Baden bei Wien and also tried other Austrian *Kurorte* as well as regularly staying in the Bohemian spas of Karlsbad, Marienbad, Franzensbad and Teplitz. In 1812 he was prescribed a tour round all four of these watering places, prompting him to write:

> I have too much of several things, of bathing, idling and so forth ... my doctor chases me from one spot to another to enable me finally to recover good health ... I must now refrain from writing any more and instead I must splash about again in the water. Hardly have I performed the duty of filling my inside with a large quantity of this water when I must have my outer surface washed down with it several times. (Anderson 1961: 1, 384)

Although he had mixed feelings about these cures, Beethoven seems on the whole to have felt they were doing him good and persisted in taking them every year throughout his life. Baden bei Wien attracted him as much for its countryside as for the waters. He took long solitary walks every morning, taking with him bundles of folded music paper on which he would scribble phrases and melodies which came to him. His favourite walk was through the Helenental valley to the west of Baden and up its thickly wooded steep slopes to the romantic ruins of the thirteenth-century Rauhenstein castle. The path through the valley following the course of the Schwechat River is now known as the Beethovenweg. He found the atmosphere of the spa conducive to creativity and composed several significant works during his stays there, including substantial parts of his Ninth Symphony in 1823.

When he came on what would be his last trip to Baden, which lasted from early May to mid-October 1825, Beethoven was in a particularly bad way with acute intestinal inflammation and subject to severe dietary restrictions from his doctor, who told him: 'no wine, no coffee; no spices of any kind ... I'll wager that if you take a drink of spirits, you'll be lying weak and exhausted on your back in a few hours.' In a letter to a friend soon after his arrival, he gave characteristically graphic details of his symptoms while expressing frustration at these restrictions:

> Still very weak and belching and so forth. I am inclined to think that I now require a stronger medicine, but it must not be constipating – Surely I might be allowed to take white wine diluted with water, for that poisonous beer is bound to make me feel sick – my catarrhal condition is showing the following symptoms, that is to say, I spit a good deal of blood, but probably only from my windpipe. But I have frequent nose bleedings, which I often had last winter as well. And there is no doubt that my stomach has become dreadfully weak, and so has, generally speaking, my whole constitution. Judging by what I know of my own constitution, my strength will hardly be restored unaided. (Anderson 1961: 3, 1195)

Beethoven closed this grim and graphic account of his symptoms with a plea set to music: '*Doktor sperrt das Tor dem Tod! Note hilft auch aus der Noth*' (Doctor close the door to death! Music will also help in need). There followed further tirades against his doctor for telling him to eat asparagus, which caused severe diarrhoea, and complaints that 'since yesterday I have eaten nothing but soup and a couple of eggs and have drunk only water; my tongue is quite yellow; and without bowel motions and tonics my stomach will never be cured.' Despite his poor physical state, he managed during this stay to compose the slow third movement of his String Quartet in A minor, Opus 132. He wrote on the score:

'*Heiliger Dankgesang eines Genesenen an die Gottheit*' (An invalid's
hymn of thanksgiving to God on his convalescence). Musicologists
have pointed out that it portrays the experience of healing and
recovery in a way not found in any other works by Beethoven
or his predecessors, through the use of the Lydian mode and the
creation of a chorale melody that serves as a basic prayer and
is then elaborated in variations. It stands as a heartfelt musical
tribute to the therapeutic benefits of spas.

Beethoven was a more serious spa-goer than many of his
contemporaries. He resisted most of the more decadent distractions
that the *Kurorte* offered, preferring rather to devote himself to his
prescribed treatments and to the healthy pursuit of long country
walks. He did not dance, he did not socialise very much, he drank
only moderately and he certainly did not gamble – in the words
of his biographer Alexander Thayer, 'he does not appear to have
known one playing-card from another.' He did, however, succumb
to two of the besetting temptations of the long-term *Kurgast*, falling
into gloomy introspective obsession with illness and death and
experiencing his own *Kurschatten*. There were at least two occasions
when he apparently became obsessed with young ladies whom he
met at spas. The first occurred during his first well-documented
visit to Baden in 1804 when his friend Franz Ries found 'a handsome
young woman sitting on the sofa with him'. Beethoven asked Ries
to play some love music, first 'Something melancholy!' and then,
'Something passionate!' The lady got up and left and Ries was
amazed to find that Beethoven had no idea who she was:

> We followed her in order to discover her lodgings. We saw her
> from a distance but suddenly she disappeared ... Beethoven
> said: 'I must find out who she is and you must help me.' A long
> time afterwards I met her in Vienna and discovered that she was
> the mistress of a foreign prince. I reported the intelligence to
> Beethoven but never heard anything more about her either from
> him or anybody else. (Forbes 1967: 354)

The other *Kurschatten* episode occurred in 1811 during a six-week stay taking the waters at Teplitz when Beethoven met the lady who seems to have come closest to being the love of his life – someone, as he later told a friend in Baden, 'a union with whom he would have considered the greatest happiness of his life'. Back in Teplitz in 1812, he wrote a tortured and confused letter pouring out his passionate feelings for 'my Immortal Beloved' and seeming at one and the same time to offer undying love and the possibility of a lifetime together and to signal a renunciation of any further attempt to marry or form a lasting relationship. The only letter in the whole of his surviving correspondence to use the affectionate form '*Du*' rather than the more formal '*Sie*', it was never posted. Whether the 'Immortal Beloved' to whom Beethoven wrote from Teplitz was the same lady whom he had first met there the previous year, and fondly recalled much later in Baden, we will never know. It is, however, significant that spas provided the backdrop to two of the apparently more significant if fleeting encounters in his troubled love life.

Beethoven was not the only early nineteenth-century European cultural giant to experience *der Kurschatten* in the spas of Bohemia. Goethe pursued several amorous adventures, first in Karlsbad (see page 122) and later in Marienbad where his virility and sexual energy were apparently greatly fortified by drinking copiously from the Ambrose Spring, known as the 'Love Spring' for its effect on both men and women. On his first visit to Marienbad in 1821, at the age of seventy-two, he developed an infatuation with the seventeen-year-old Ulrike von Levetzow and became her regular companion on walks, at tea parties and at balls over three successive summer seasons there. In 1823, he proposed to her. Ulrike, who had thought of him as a grandfather-like figure, was flustered and gave him a non-committal answer. Her mother took more decisive action and whisked her away to Karlsbad. Goethe was devastated, pouring out his feelings of despair and desolation in his famous 'Marienbad Elegy', which he composed in the coach as he left the town. It later became part of his *Trilogy of Passion*, which also celebrated the musical talents of a young Polish pianist and composer, Maria Szymanowska, with whom he had become infatuated in Marienbad. He sent another intense poem, beginning 'Passion brings suffering', to a third lady who seems to have captivated him there. After his rejection by Ulrike, he never returned to the Bohemian spas which had been such an important part of his life. It has been calculated that he spent a total of 1,114 days (just over three years) in them over a period of thirty-eight years. Ulrike never married and lived as a spinster to the age of ninety-five.

Frédéric Chopin also came under the *Kurschatten* spell seemingly exerted by the spas of West Bohemia. He spent twenty-three days with his parents in Karlsbad in the summer of 1835, which were among the happiest of his life, principally because he fell in love there with the daughter of a Polish general, to whom he dedicated two mazurkas. The following year he joined another Polish family for four weeks in Marienbad and became infatuated with the daughter, Maria. Her mother put a stop to the relationship. When his correspondence with Maria was found after his death, the words 'my grief' were scribbled on top of the bundle of letters.

Augustus Granville visited Karlsbad just a year after Chopin as part of his general tour of mid-European spas. He gave a graphic description of the springs, which were thronged at five in the morning with drinkers assisted by local girls, 'the little nymphs of the *Sprudel*', equipped with four-foot-long poles with a cup holder at one end, who plunged their beakers into 'the smoking column of water'. Meanwhile excellent bands played music by Beethoven and Rossini, 'enlivening the dull and dispirited, cheering the discouraged and the hypochondriacs'. He noted the very aristocratic clientele but was also struck how most people were there for the purpose of health rather than amusement, spending five to six weeks on their cure and taking it very seriously. Amusements were provided to alleviate the boredom of the cure, including ventriloquists, Tyrolean minstrels, rope-dancers, Indian jugglers and fire-kings, but overall Granville felt Karlsbad's serious therapeutic focus fully justified its designation as the Hospital of Europe. He found a similar atmosphere in Marienbad, which he noted was especially renowned for treating melancholic indigestion, a condition particularly affecting men aged between thirty-five and forty. Granville was impressed by the gas baths there where patients sat in wooden cupboards on stools perforated with holes through which carbon dioxide piped from underground worked its wonders on their legs and bottoms. Overall, he was taken by Marienbad's sober and restrained atmosphere:

> The greatest simplicity of manners, regularity of hours, and the strictest propriety of conduct on all hands, seem to be the order of the day. Here are no gaming tables – no facilities for intrigue – and few temptations to attract the mere lounger, the idler and the rogue ... Marienbad is not a spa of pleasure. It is a lovely and enchanting retreat for invalids. (Granville 2012: 129)

Baden-Baden, another port of call on Granville's 1836 tour of European spas, provoked a rather different reaction. He gave careful and detailed descriptions of the springs and the baths, noting that 'a Baden warm bath is exciting and two of them in one day would be productive of dangerous irritation' and that 'much mischief has arisen from its indiscriminate adoption'. He cited the case of a rich merchant found dead in his bath one evening and a lady who had lost the use of her limbs after taking three hot baths. His overall impression, however, was of the prevailing emphasis on amusement rather than health and the low morals of many of the *Kurgäste*. He was distressed by the number of young Englishwomen frequenting the casino and hanging on the arms of elderly German men and by the wild and libidinous character of the evening dances. He was especially disturbed by the sight of an exquisitely elegant married English lady who would 'at the slightest invitation from a booted hussar, or an embroidered *attachi*, or a disguised *vaurien* from the lower class, plunge with them into all the attitudes, now violent and now languishing, of a dance better suited for Bacchanalian or Andalusian representation'. Her wild abandon particularly concerned the sensitive doctor as he recognised the 'deep round flush of consumption' on her 'alabaster and shining cheek' (Granville 2012: 33).

Granville's observations confirm that health, hedonism and hypochondria continued to intermingle as key ingredients in the appeal of spas throughout the nineteenth century. Health remained important and its profile was raised with the continuing professionalisation of those practising medicine and the emergence of balneotherapy (treatment of diseases by bathing in and drinking from mineral springs) as a distinct medical speciality. Two professional bodies devoted to medical hydrology were established in France in 1853, and a bi-monthly magazine, *Gazette des Eaux*, started appearing five years later. In Germany, a *Handbuch der Balneotherapie*, first published in 1861, reached its seventh edition by 1867 and a Balneology Society was founded in Berlin in 1878. The cure was still at the centre of the spas' *raison d'être* and doctors remained ubiquitous and significant figures in *Kurorte* and *villes d'eaux* – as Guy de Maupassant put it in *Mont-Oriol*, 'in watering places doctors seem to rise out of the springs as naturally as gas bubbles.'

A huge variety of conditions were regarded as susceptible to successful treatment through balneotherapy. Granville's list of the disorders 'in which the Gastein water has evinced its marvelous power' was typically comprehensive and eclectic:

Depression of spirits and general languor of the constitution, from anxiety of mind – paralysis, in young as well as aged people, consequent on repeated rheumatism, gout, or apoplectic attacks, and such as is produced by irregularities of every sort – affections of the spine – hysteric attacks, and other sufferings owing to sexual disturbance in females – erotic diseases, imperfectly cured – contractions in the muscles of the limbs, or in the joints, and hip disease – premature old age – chronic ulcers or eruptions – derangement of the digestive organs, accompanied

by laxity or inactivity of the stomach, or following obstinate
diarrhoea and dysentery. (Granville 2012: 86)

Although it is mentioned in the above list, along with the intriguing
'imperfectly cured erotic diseases', gout did not assume the same
importance in the nineteenth century as it had in the eighteenth.
There was still an emphasis in spa medicine on diseases brought on
by over-indulgence and sedentary and over-intellectual lifestyles.
Granville noted that the main conditions treated at Karlsbad were
'gluttony, and high living, immoderate potation of strong liquors,
violent exercise of the body, intense thought and violent mental
excitement' (Granville 2012: 113). The quest to cure obesity
became an increasingly common reason for people to come to spas.
Visiting the baths at Leuk in Switzerland in 1878, Mark Twain saw
'the largest lady I had ever seen'. She was there 'to get rid of her
extra flesh'. He was later able to report that 'five weeks of soaking
– five uninterrupted hours of it every day – had accomplished
her purpose and reduced her to the right proportions' (Twain
1996: 394). During a stay in Buxton the following year, Edward
Bradbury was struck by the sight of 'a very gross and corpulent
man in a bath chair being pulled by a pale man, consumptive and
shrunken', leading him to observe 'Bath-chair men are generally
pale and shrunken, and their fares fat and ruddy' (Langham and
Wells 2005: 92). Alongside weight reduction, the promotion of
female fertility and male virility continued to feature prominently
in lists of spa cures. The desire to conceive led several prominent
women to take the waters, with some, like Joséphine Bonaparte
in Plombières, gaining no benefit and others, like the Archduchess
Sophie in Ischl, finding them very efficacious. The enhancement
of male potency remained a major selling point for several spas.
A physician at Aix-les-Bains confidently asserted in 1862: 'It is
well known that sulfurous waters in general, and, more notably
the springs in Aix, augment the body's vital forces and, typically,
elevate the erectability of the penis' (Mackaman 1998: 101). Spas

also offered cures for those whose penises might have been rather too erect too many times. Gustave Flaubert made several visits to Vichy in the early 1860s ostensibly for the sake of his mother's health but in fact almost certainly in an attempt to cure the venereal disease he had contracted from prostitutes, both male and female, on his travels in the Levant.

Those taking cures as a more general tonic and pick-me-up were often struck by the fact that the healthy and the hypochondriacs outnumbered the genuinely ill. During a cure at Karlsbad in 1843, in which he was prescribed a daily dose of seven goblets of water, the seventh Earl of Shaftesbury noted in his diary:

> Felt half ashamed to drink them in my comparatively vigorous health, but really one need not entertain such delicate conceptions. Saw robust and muscular men, in full swig, who could sustain or undertake a siege, walk or eat for a wager. Took courage and affected as much necessity as they did. Baths and springs exhibit very few apparently sickly people. Seem bent on society and dissipation quite as much as on cure. (Hodder 1892: 270)

Shaftesbury was sceptical about the effects of his drinking cure which he described as 'the life of a whale' and observed that 'the waters seem to produce on me neither good nor evil; a hogshead of the Thames would be quite as effective.'

A significant change took place in many spas during the nineteenth century which probably explains why visitors like Shaftesbury saw very few seriously ill people around. The very sick were increasingly shut away and separated from other cure guests. In part, this was a consequence of the replacement of communal by individual baths and the introduction of new more specialised treatments, like inhalations, which were carried out in private rooms. The tendency of spas to specialise in certain areas of medicine led to some focusing almost entirely on the seriously ill. These were often remotely sited and largely shunned by those seeking the more decadent attractions and diversions of spa life. This trend was particularly apparent in the North American spas. Virginia's Hot Springs developed such a reputation for invalidism that stage coaches drove directly past its hotels without stopping and the few healthy travellers who did stop there became 'quite disgusted with the place' (Chambers 2002: 73).

The sick could not be completely hidden away and they were still to be found in the more fashionable spas. A guide to Vichy published in 1836 felt it wise to warn visitors that while most guests there would enjoy eating and talking, there would inevitably be 'a small number of individuals whose health does not permit them to engage in either of these functions' and whose presence 'could diminish the gaiety of the table' (Mackaman 1998: 3). A visitor to Red Sulphur Springs in Virginia in 1839 was put off by the constant coughing and spitting of his fellow guests and complained 'one can't divest oneself of the idea of consumptive disease even at meals' (Chambers 2002: 74). There were other indications that the sick were increasingly being seen as something of an embarrassment and a drag on the amusements and diversions which were becoming the main attractions of many spas. On the whole, those staying in the grander spas were not too bothered by invalids, who tended to be up early to take the waters and not around late at night for the balls, concerts and gambling sessions. French doctors advised those genuinely ill and taking a cure to fight 'the great temptation to join the social circle' and 'to frequent the salon as little as possible in the evenings' (Mackaman 1998: 102).

This trend towards the sick becoming a hidden minority in spas is borne out by statistics. From 1850 French *villes d'eaux* counted separately those following a course of medically prescribed treatment (*curistes*) and those essentially coming for pleasure, diversion and general relaxation (*touristes*). In Aix-les-Bains in 1861 the former still outnumbered the latter by 4,000 to 2,500 but by 1880 the roles had been reversed: there were 13,000 *touristes* and only 6,500 *curistes*, and by 1911 the ratio was 30,000 *touristes* to 11,000 *curistes*.

Royal and imperial patronage continued to be important in putting the main European spas on the map. This was especially true of Ischl in Austria, to whose waters the emperor Franz Joseph seemingly owed his very existence. Ischl (the official *Bad* designation did not come until 1906 but it was recognised as a leading spa before then), which nestles along the banks of the River Traun in the middle of the mountainous Salzkammergut (salt chamber) region of Upper Austria, was for long a small and unremarkable town in which most people made a living from forestry or salt mining. In 1820 Dr Josef Götz, a resident physician, discovered that adding water from the local hot sulphur springs to the brine baths taken by the workers in the salt mines helped to ease their rheumatism and skin complaints. He recommended them to Dr Wirer, physician to the imperial court, who publicised their therapeutic properties and commended them specifically to Sophie, wife of Archduke Franz Karl, on whom hopes for the Habsburg succession rested but who seemed unable to bear children. In 1828, after suffering several miscarriages, she responded to Dr Wirer's suggestion that she try the salt baths at Ischl. Sophie loved the atmosphere there which reminded her of the Bavarian mountains she knew as a girl. Eighteen months after her treatment, in August 1830, she gave birth to a healthy boy, Franz Joseph, who would reign as Austrian emperor from 1848 to 1916. Following two further treatments, she gave birth to another two sons. The three brothers became known as the salt princes.

Franz Joseph went on to spend eighty-three of his eighty-six summers in Ischl. His parents, not surprisingly, found the place enchanting and established it as their main summer base. They first took him there in July 1831 when he was just one to escape a cholera-ridden Vienna. Ascending to the imperial throne at the age of eighteen, he established an annual ritual of bringing the court there every summer. He would arrive early in July when the hunting season started, forsaking his Vienna residences, the Hofburg and Schönbrunn Palace, in favour of the more modest Kaiservilla set in a large park on the outskirts of the spa town, and usually stayed until his birthday on 18 August. While in Ischl, he wore leather shorts, green jacket, thick woollen socks, mountaineer's boots and a Tyrolean hat and devoted himself with an almost fanatical passion to hunting and shooting, killing a total of 50,556 birds and animals during his stays there. His tally included 18,031 pheasants, 2,051 chamois, 1,442 wild boar and 1,436 stags.

Throughout Franz Joseph's reign Ischl became a magnet for the crowned heads and high society of Europe and beyond. King Wilhelm I of Prussia, later emperor of Germany, visited several times, as did the emperor of Brazil and the kings of Britain, Denmark, Rumania, Serbia, Greece, Bulgaria and Siam. With the imperial family and their royal guests came aristocrats, politicians, artists, composers, writers and the inevitable hangers-on. Ischl provided several of its distinguished guests with *Kurschatten*, mostly drawn from the ranks of the singers and actresses performing there for the summer season. Franz Joseph had his own rather unusual one, the actress Katharina Schratt, whom he had much admired on stage. It was actually his wife, Elisabeth, whom he had first met and become engaged to in Ischl, who seems to have engineered and promoted their relationship. Feeling guilty about the effects of her withdrawal from court life into a lonely exile, she set up the actress as a companion for the husband she could no longer live with or love. In 1889, Katharina bought a villa in Ischl close to the imperial summer residence. Elisabeth suggested giving her a key to a little secret door through which she could directly access the garden of the Kaiservilla without going through the streets of the town. Actress and emperor went on to spend much time together and their close relationship continued after Elisabeth's assassination at the hands of an anarchist in 1898.

Among other visitors to Ischl who succumbed to *Kurschatten* while there was Nikolaus Lenau, widely regarded as Austria's greatest lyric poet and often compared to Byron. He became totally infatuated with Caroline Unger, an Austrian contralto best remembered as the soloist at the first performance of Beethoven's

Ninth Symphony in 1824 who had turned the deaf composer round so that he could see the audience's applause and appreciation at the end of the work. They had an intense affair and became briefly engaged but it ended in tears and Lenau died broken-hearted at the age of forty-eight. Perhaps the most unlikely *Kurschatten* experience in Ischl occurred in 1865 as the result of a chance meeting in front of the Hotel Post between the ultra-conservative Prussian statesman, Otto von Bismarck, and the glamorous soprano Pauline Lucca. After some flirtatious banter she talked him into accompanying her to a photographer's studio. Bismarck's adoring gaze and the proximity of his knee to hers made the resulting photograph a sensation and led his political opponents to mock the future Iron Chancellor's reputation as a severe and devoutly pious Lutheran. He had the original negative destroyed and tried to buy up all existing copies of the photograph.

Vichy developed as the Queen of the French spas thanks largely to royal patronage. The Parc Thermal was laid out on the personal orders of Emperor Napoleon I in 1812. Napoleon III assured the prosperity of the town by taking cures for his rheumatism and gout on five occasions in the 1860s, usually staying for twenty-five days under close medical supervision. Following his first visit, he ordered the construction of a town hall, church, train station and casino. On subsequent visits, he settled with his suite in specially built Swiss-style chalets, which can still be seen today. He rose at 7 a.m. for his first bath and then went for a walk before taking his first glass of water at the Célestins source. Other aspects of his cure regime were rather less severe – a typical dinner menu consisted of soup, salmon trout, gigot of lamb, plum pudding and dessert of fruit and cheese followed by coffee and liqueurs – but he did eschew balls, concerts and soirées. His final cure in 1865 was terminated abruptly when he left after only eleven days. The official explanation was that a political crisis necessitated his return to Paris but the real reason was the poor state of his health. He was apparently liked by the locals who regarded him as 'a natural dreamer, or rather a melancholic' (Vauthey 1984: 28). A bust of Napoleon III, installed in 1991 in the park that bears his name, has an inscription with his words 'I am more pleased here than anywhere else, for this is my creation.' His wife, Eugénie, was similarly enthusiastic about taking the waters and has a source named after her.

Several of the most fashionable German spas benefited from the attentions of monarchs and emperors. King Wilhelm I of Prussia (from 1871, as Kaiser Wilhelm, the first German emperor) was a huge enthusiast for spa cures, patronising Bad Homburg, where he famously walked through the *Kurpark* snapping his fingers at trees which he did not like and which were subsequently felled, and Bad Ems, to which he made twenty visits, staying in relatively modest quarters in what became known as the Kaiserflügel, the east wing of the old *Kurhaus* which is now Häcker's Grand Hotel. Bad Ems was also favoured by Tsar Alexander II who went there for four years running in the 1870s. The presence of the two men can still be felt in the town today. A commanding statue of Wilhelm I, uncharacteristically dressed in civilian clothes rather than a uniform, stands at the end of the *Kurpark* looking down on a modest bust of the tsar. Both men also left an ecclesiastical legacy: the Kaiser Wilhelm Church near the station, built to provide a more central place of Protestant worship than the existing church at the end of the village, and the magnificent Russian Orthodox church on the riverfront, consecrated in 1876 in the presence of both kaiser and tsar. There were also Russian Orthodox churches in Bad Homburg, Wiesbaden, Wildbad and Baden-Baden, a testament to the huge popularity of German *Kurorte* with the Russians who for much of the mid- and later nineteenth century were the largest group of foreign guests in terms of nationality. In Bad Ems's peak year of popularity (1871), for example, there were 1,077 Russian *Kurgäste*, along with 955 English, 538 Dutch, 336 Belgians, 260 Americans and 203 French.

It was the patronage of Germany's chancellor rather than its monarch that substantially raised the profile of the leading *Kurort* in Bavaria, Bad Kissingen. Bismarck regularly visited it from the early 1870s in an effort to counter the effects of his very unhealthy lifestyle, which involved seven-course dinners, heavy drinking at all meals plus as much as two bottles of champagne in the afternoon, and chain smoking – he even devised a multipronged holder so he could have three Havana cigars on the go at once. Not surprisingly, he suffered from a combination of insomnia, haemorrhoids, stomach pains, indigestion, gout and nervous irritability. Staying in a private apartment in Bad Kissingen, he walked to the *Kurhaus* every morning along a route heavily guarded by local police (although this did not stop an assassination attempt in 1874), bathed in private and then returned in a carriage supplied by King Ludwig II of Bavaria. His stays there seemed to have had a beneficial effect and he claimed that he owed his good health 'to a loving God and the healing waters of Bad Kissingen'.

Baden-Baden established its reputation as the most fashionable of the German *Kurorte* partly on the basis of its numerous royal visitors, most notably Kaiser Wilhelm I who spent forty summers there, always arriving with twelve black horses and twelve coachmen and staying in the Hotel Messmer, which changed its name to Maison Messmer during his residence as protocol forbade the emperor from staying in a hotel. Tsar Alexander II lived in similar splendour during his stays there and Napoleon III lodged at the spacious Villa Stéphanie. By contrast, Queen Victoria, who found the air 'so becoming', occupied three modest rooms in a small wooden house belonging to a relative, Prince von Hohenlohe. Other royal *Kurgäste* at Baden-Baden included King Alfonso XIII of Spain, the emperors of Siam and Brazil and several kings of Norway and Sweden. As well as enhancing the atmosphere of exclusivity and grandeur, the town's royal visitors also attracted scandal and conspiracy. A visiting Russian prince was killed by his mistress and Prince Stourdza of Romania was assassinated by a group of anarchists disguised as priests.

Baden-Baden had conspicuously elegant and opulent premises for balneotherapy. A magnificent *Trinkhalle* was built in 1842, fronted with sixteen massive Corinthian columns and a long gallery with murals showing local legends and stories. It now houses the Tourist Information Centre and a fountain from which visitors can still drink the piping-hot water. The main bathing establishment, the Friedrichsbad, opened in 1877 and was designed to emulate the ancient baths of Diocletian and Caracalla in Rome, offering thermal water baths at varying temperatures, vapour baths, hot-air baths, mud baths, douches, electric baths, grape-and-milk cures and compressed-air chambers. Several of the grand hotels had their own bath houses and there were also private sanatoria. Walks were laid out around the town for those taking the 'Terrainkur'. A visiting English medical practitioner described Baden-Baden as 'a sort of invalid's compendium, where various kinds of physical and other treatments can be applied in addition to the treatment by the thermal waters' (Yeo 1904: 82).

It was not so much its medical facilities as its social ambience, glamour and elegance that really accounted for the popularity of Baden-Baden. Eugène Guinot, society editor of the French newspaper Le Siècle, observed in 1845: 'in Europe there are two capitals, Paris for the winter and Baden-Baden for the summer.' In 1857, when for the first time the number of overseas Kurgäste, coming mostly from Russia, France and England, exceeded 50,000, the New York Times dubbed it 'the Boulevard of Europe'. A guide to mineral springs and climatic resorts across the world noted that 'the hotel and other accommodation probably exceeds that of any other town in Europe and amusements and distractions of all kinds are provided' (Yeo 1904: 80). Chief among these amusements and distractions was gambling. The earliest official mention of licensed gambling in Baden-Baden is in 1748. In 1809, a gaming room was opened in the Konversationshaus on the Market Square (now the Town Hall). In 1824, a Kurhaus was built with designated gambling rooms. King Louis Philippe's decision in 1838 to close all gaming houses in France gave a huge boost to Baden-Baden as Frenchmen flocked across the border to play the tables there, with roulette taking over from card games as the main attraction. From 1838 the casino was managed by Jacques Bénazet, who had previously run the Palais Royal in Paris. He and his son Edouard, who took over after his father's death in 1848, invested huge sums in the casino. Between 1854 and 1858 four new gaming rooms were built on to the side of the *Kurhaus*. Decorated with gilded stucco, extravagant red plush and massive chandeliers, they were also used for theatrical productions and balls (Plate 8).

Edouard Bénazet considerably enhanced the facilities and the elegance of Baden-Baden. He built a large theatre in 1862 designed by the Paris architect Séchan in the style of the Paris Opera. He also substantially endowed the town's first Protestant church, surely one of the few places of worship to have been built out of the profits of a casino. His greatest contribution was in laying out the grounds around the Lichtentaler Allee, a path that runs along the banks of the River Oos and connects Baden-Baden with the thirteenth-century Cistercian Abbey at Lichtental, 2.3 kilometres (1.4 miles) away. In the seventeenth century the ground around the path had been planted with oak trees. Bénazet developed it as an elegant promenade, turning the first stretch, starting from behind his theatre, into an English-style park with fountains shaded by oaks and beeches. Further along, he created a more formal French garden and beyond it a broad avenue lined by lime trees with meadows alongside. Elegant hotels and villas were built along the Allee, their gardens running down to the clear shallow waters of the Oos. The Lichtentaler Allee became the centre of Baden-Baden social life, the place in which to engage in the favourite activity of *Kurgäste*, to see and to be seen.

We can gain a very vivid impression of the ambience of Baden-Baden at the height of its popularity, and not least of its more hidden shadow side, from the writings of the four leading Russian novelists who took cures there in the middle of the nineteenth century. Between them, they highlight key areas of its appeal, with Nikolai Gogol focusing on health and himself epitomising hypochondria, Ivan Turgenev experiencing and describing the classic *Kurschatten* experience, and both Leo Tolstoy and Fyodor Dostoyevsky falling victim to and writing about addiction to its gaming tables.

Gogol had been a hypochondriac from boyhood, obsessed with his health and his physical imperfections. He had the archetypal hypochondriacal combination of gout, haemorrhoids and oscillating constipation and diarrhoea, not helped by a sedentary lifestyle and over-indulgence. A modern diagnosis of his condition would probably be irritable bowel syndrome. Told by his doctor that taking the water at Baden-Baden was the best way to cure his manifold complaints, he dutifully went there four times between 1836 and 1844, benefiting not just from the waters but also from a strict diet and exercise regime. He felt himself in a minority in being there largely to take a cure and not to engage in more frivolous activities, noting that there was no one there who was seriously ill and that most had come simply to enjoy themselves. His attention to the serious business of the cure paid off; he obtained some relief from his symptoms and found that the regime stimulated his creative muse.

Tolstoy came to Baden-Baden in 1857. Unlike Gogol, he was in reasonable health, apart from the gonorrhea that he had contracted as a student and regularly topped up with one-night stands, and had no interest in taking the waters. What drew him, like so many others, was the casino. He made a beeline for the roulette tables on his first evening and spent most of his time at them, playing straight through the day from morning until evening. He lost disastrously, borrowing money from friends and relations only to gamble it all away. He was desperate and never returned after this first disastrous visit. He put his experience of Baden-Baden, a place where, in his words, 'a glittering façade masked inner decadence', into two of his novels. The first, *Family Happiness* (1859), describes the newly married Masha Alexandrovna spending a summer in Baden-Baden. Left unchaperoned, she very nearly commits adultery with a much older but very dashing Italian adventurer who attempts to seduce her. There is a pervasive atmosphere throughout the novel of the shadow side of spa life. Nothing is quite what it seems and Masha comes to realise that everything she had enjoyed about Baden-Baden turns out on reflection to have been illusory, and pertain only to the surface. A similar sense underlies his treatment of Bad Soden, an actual spa but almost certainly based on Baden-Baden, in *Anna Karenina*, where, as we have seen, Prince Shcherbátsky is struck by the 'monstrous contrast' between the music, the gambling and the desperately sick and dying people and feels it a sad, sad place (see page 35).

Turgenev first came to Baden-Baden in 1857 in response to a desperate plea for help from his friend Tolstoy. He initially made the mistake of handing him a large wad of notes, which were blown in an hour at the roulette tables. Whereas Tolstoy returned to Russia, never to return, Turgenev came back to Baden-Baden in 1863, making it his home for the next six years. His reason for moving there was to be near his close friend, the French soprano Pauline Viardot-García, who had moved there with her husband from Paris. It has often been suggested that Turgenev and Pauline were lovers. The guide who took me round Baden-Baden even thought they had an illegitimate child. He certainly contributed to her salons and basked in the reflected glory of her glittering image. Soon after arriving there he was afflicted with an inflamed prostate, which he told a friend, meant 'no good thinking of shooting or champagne or crumpet – though as far as this last is concerned, the devil can take it' (Schapiro 1978: 193). He was captivated by the atmosphere of the place, writing to Flaubert in 1865: 'Do come to Baden-Baden. Here are the most magnificent trees I have ever seen. They do wonders for the eyes and the soul.' He does not seem to have tried taking the waters, even when he was diagnosed with gout. This was initially misdiagnosed as a heart attack and he was warned again to abstain from meat and wine and have 'no dallying with the fairer sex'. However, he ignored this advice, as he had before, and continued to enjoy Baden-Baden's glittering atmosphere and the company of Pauline. He eventually left when she and her husband moved to London on the outbreak of the Franco-Prussian War in 1870.

Baden-Baden was the setting for Turgenev's novel *Smoke*, written between 1865 and 1866 and published in 1867. Its opening sequence, set in front of the Konversationshaus, perfectly captures the atmosphere of the *Kurort* with its motley collection of 'Italians, Moldavians, American spiritualists, smart secretaries of foreign embassies, and Germans of effeminate, but prematurely circumspect physiognomy' together with the Russian aristocrats who congregate around the 'Russian Tree' in the *Kurpark* (Turgenev 1906: 5–6). The book's central character, Grigory Mikhailovich Litvinov, a young Russian farmer, finds himself in Baden-Baden because his fiancée's aunt, Kapitolina Markovna Shestov, despite being a fierce democrat and opponent of aristocracy, 'could not resist the temptation of gazing for once on this fashionable society'. It is clear that this is what attracts people – as one Russian general comments, 'One doesn't, as a rule, come to Baden for the waters' (Turgenev 1906: 12, 136).

The plot is a familiar one involving *Kurschatten*, in this case Litvinov's disastrous seduction by the older femme fatale, Irina, who is married to a Russian general. Baden-Baden plays a key role in this story. As the title implies, it is portrayed as being all smoke and shadow, a kind of make-believe, enchanted place where what is half a dream and half a nightmare is played out. Litvinov experiences there 'some sensation unknown before … strong, sweet and evil. His self-confidence had vanished, and his peace of mind had vanished too, and his respect for himself; of his former spiritual condition nothing was left.' This tendency of spa life to strip away one's moral consciousness is also shown by the usually moralistic and matronly Kapitolina Markovna's reaction to the gaming tables with their spinning roulette wheels, quickly moving croupiers' scoops and heaps of gold, which put her in 'a sort of speechless stupor; she altogether forgot that she ought to feel moral indignation, and could only gaze and gaze. The whizz of the ivory ball into the bottom of the roulette thrilled her to the marrow of her bones.' Eventually, the spell is broken. Kapitolina beseeches Litvinov to abandon the temptress Irina and return to his wholesome fiancée: 'Leave this

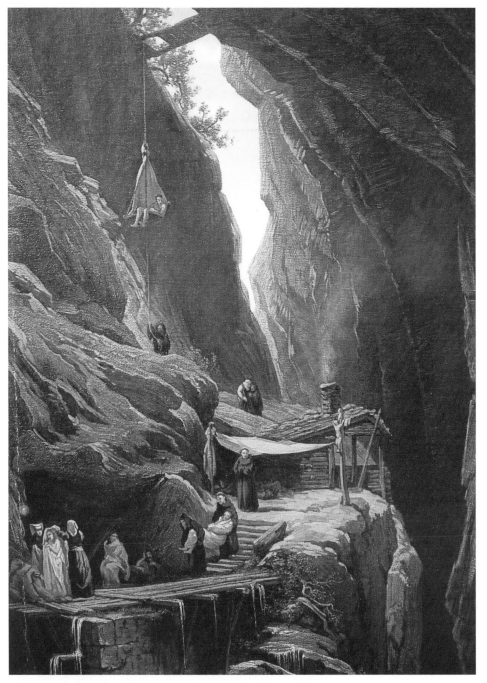

1 The original baths at Pfäfers in the Tamina Gorge.

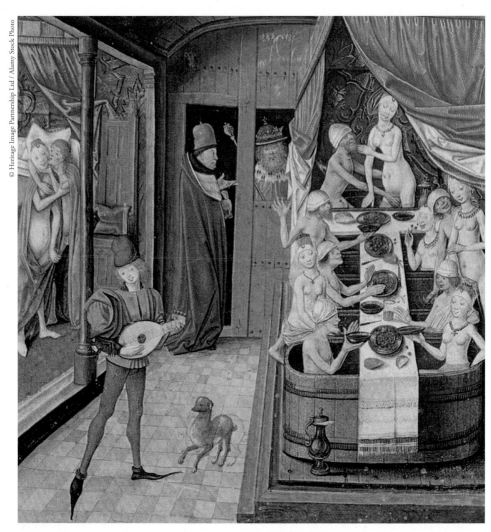

2 A Bathhouse. From Facta et dicta memorabilia by Valerius
Maximus, c 1470. Artist: Master of Anthony of Burgundy.

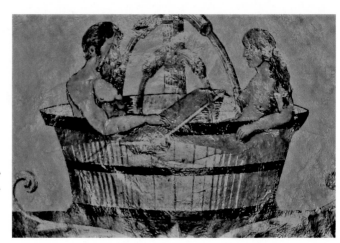

3 Coat of arms,
Baden bei Wien.

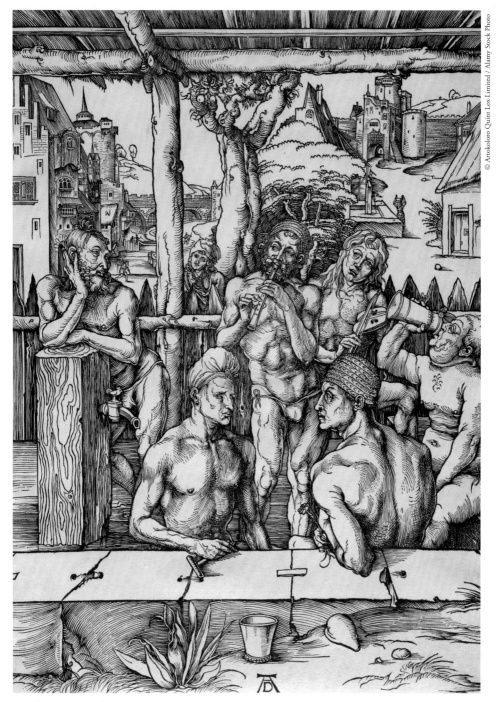

4 'The Men's Bath House' – engraving by Albrecht Dürer, c.1496.

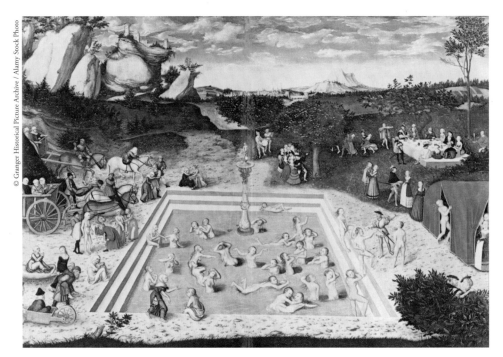

5 'The Fountain of Youth' by Lucas Cranach, the younger, 1546.

6 The Baths at Louèche, Switzerland – painting by Hans Bock, 1597.

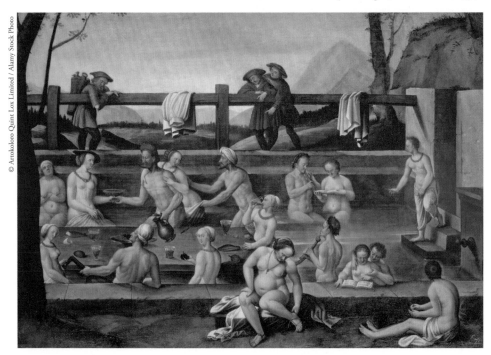

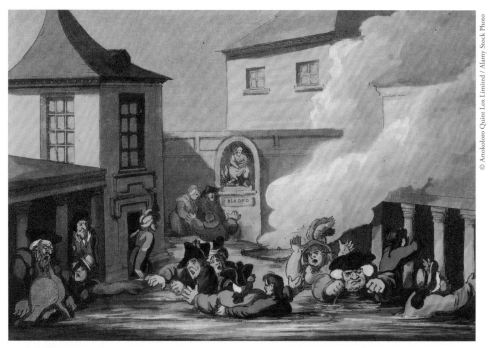

7 'The Comforts of Bath' – engraving by Thomas Rowlandson, c.1798.

8 Inside the casino, Baden-Baden.

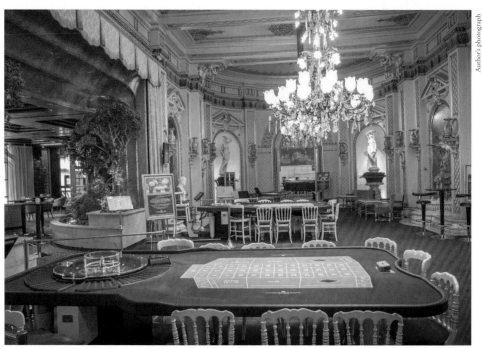

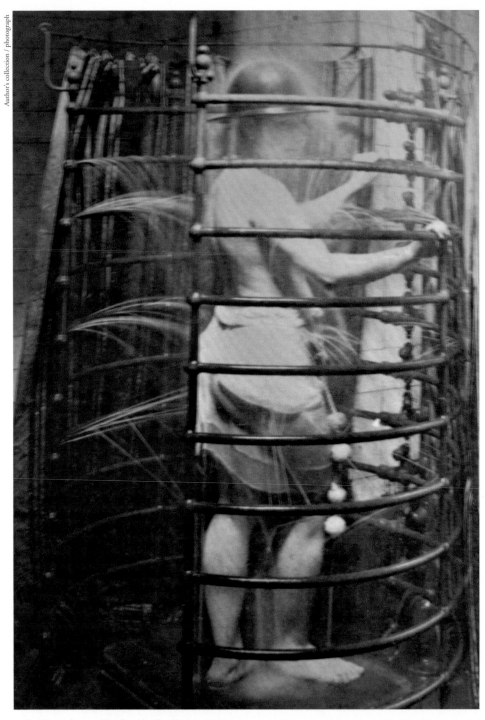

9 La Douche en Circle, Aix-les-Bains, c.1900.

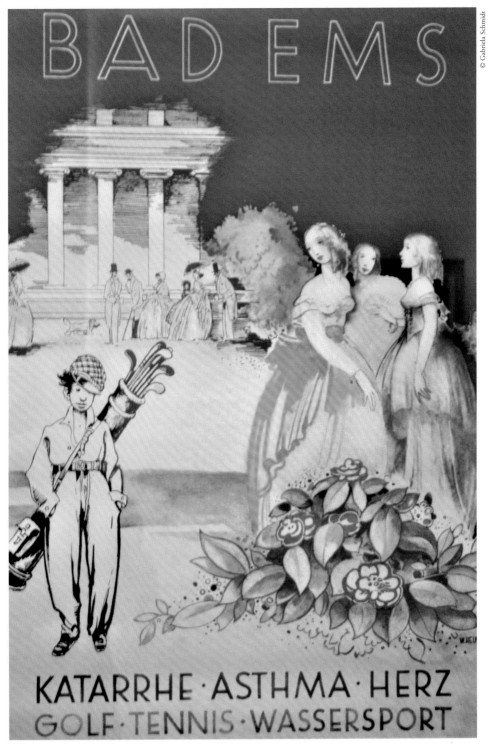

10 Poster for Bad Ems designed by Walter Heimig c. 1930.

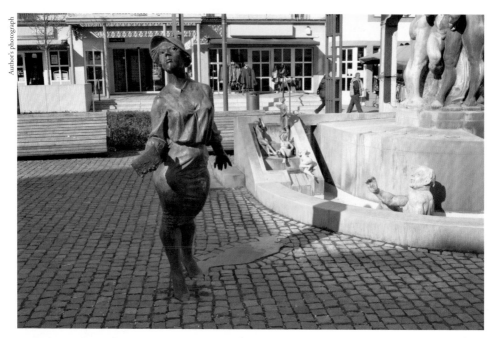

11 Der Kurschattenbrunnen in Bad Wildungen shows a young lady casting her shadow over an elderly *kurgast*.

12 Edward VII and Kaiser Franz Joseph in the Kurpark at Mariánské Lázně with one of the distinctive single seats between them.

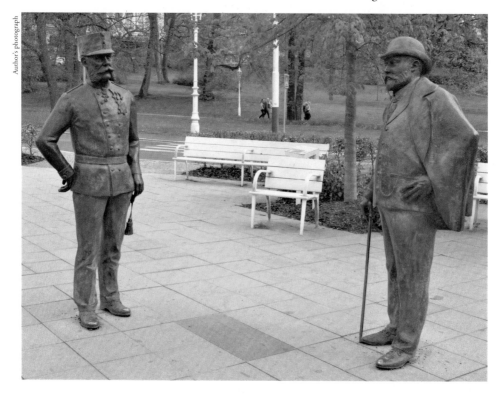

hateful Baden-Baden, let us go away together, only throw off this enchantment.' Litvinov does at last see sense and breaks the spell in which he has been held with the result that 'all that had passed in Baden appeared to him dimly as in a dream' (Turgenev 1906: 205, 211, 263, 302). There are few novels that more accurately portray the hidden shadow side of spas and the sinister power that their beguiling enchantment can exert.

Dostoyevsky, the last of the quartet of Russian novelists to come to and write about Baden-Baden, was the most addicted to and damaged by its decadent diversions, specifically the seductive allure of its roulette tables. He had first caught the spa gambling bug in 1862 on a short visit to Wiesbaden where, despite being afflicted with chronic obstructive pulmonary disease, liver complaints, epilepsy and haemorrhoids, he does not seem to have gone anywhere near the waters. He returned there the following year, leaving his dying wife in Moscow, having taken up with a much younger woman, Polina Suslova. As on his earlier trip, he managed to lose all his money, which had come in the form of a grant from the St Petersburg Society for Support of Needy Writers and Scholars. This did not stop him going on to Baden-Baden where he met and sponged off Turgenev. He was back in Wiesbaden in 1865, once again raiding the fund for supporting needy authors and working on *Crime and Punishment* as he recklessly gambled more and more. Full of self-loathing, he appealed to the ever generous Turgenev who stumped up more cash, which was promptly spent in the casino. Dostoyevsky also managed to secure an emergency loan from the town's resident Russian Orthodox priest with whom he embarked on a deep discussion about free will and charitable love that would later find its way into his novel *The Brothers Karamazov*.

Dostoyevsky's great contribution to nineteenth-century spa literature, *The Gambler*, appropriately came about out of a desperate effort to make some money quickly to pay off his gambling debts. Pressure from his creditors had forced him to sell to his publisher for 3,000 roubles all the rights to his previous books and also to an as yet unwritten one of at least 160 pages. If he failed to produce the new work by 1 November 1866, his publisher would have the right to issue everything he wrote for the next nine years without paying him a penny. A month before the deadline, he had written nothing. A friend suggested he employ a stenographer and for the next twenty-six days he sat in his room in St Petersburg from noon to 4.30 p.m. dictating a novel about obsessive gambling to the twenty-year-old Anna Grigorievna. He completed the book just in time.

The Gambler is set in the fictional German spa of Roulettenberg, which is clearly an amalgam of Wiesbaden and Baden-Baden. As the title suggests, most of the action takes place in the casino and the novel is essentially about hopeless addiction and the irreconcilability of the two passionate obsessions conceived by the narrator, Alexei Ivanovich, during a season at the spa, one being for Polina, a general's stepdaughter, and the other for roulette. He is equally in thrall to both and one of the reasons that he goes on gambling is that he thinks his winnings will impress Polina, whereas in fact his addiction repels her, in much the same way that Dostoyevsky's gambling turned off the real-life Polina Suslova when they were in Baden-Baden together. Much of the book is clearly autobiographical. As in *Smoke*, the picture painted of the life of a fashionable spa is one of shallowness, sordidness, self-deception and play-acting and there is an abiding sense that nothing and nobody are quite as they seem. Alexei reflects at one point that although the Russian newspapers rave about the magnificence of the casinos in the German *Kurorte*, in reality 'there is no splendour whatsoever in those sordid rooms' which are full of cheating, stealing and desperation. A passage towards the end has Alexei going frantically from spa to spa, with Bad Homburg, Spa and Baden-Baden all being mentioned as well as the generic and fictional Roulettenberg. He is overwhelmed with depression and reduced to 'a worse position than the meanest beggar'. Ultimately, he reflects on what it is that has driven him, encapsulating the persistent theme in the hidden history of spas that they are all about show and appearance: 'It was not the money that

I valued: what I wanted was to make all this mob of Heintzes, hotel proprietors, and fine ladies of Baden talk about me, recount my story, wonder at me, extol my doings, and worship my winnings' (Dostoyevsky 1962: 298).

As that reference to 'Heintzes' suggests, Dostoyevsky was not very keen on the Germans he encountered at the *Kurorte* to which he resorted so often. Nor did he much care for the French. Indeed, the only non-Russian character who gets any praise in *The Gambler* is an Englishman, Mr Astley. In this view, he was very much at odds with Turgenev, whose subtext in *Smoke* is the superiority of German culture over that of Russia. *Smoke* indeed caused a major falling-out between the two men. For Turgenev, critical though he was of it in many respects, Baden-Baden represented all that was best in West European culture. It was cosmopolitan, open and cultured in contrast to the brutal primitivism of his native Russia. Dostoyevsky could never forgive him for that observation and they had a major row in Baden-Baden in 1867. Despite his dislike of the German *Kurorte* and all that they represented, Dostoyevsky went on visiting and gambling in them for another five years after the publication of *The Gambler*. He was back in Baden-Baden in 1867 with Anna Grigorievna, whom he had married shortly after dictating the book to her. They spent a disastrous five-week honeymoon there, with him having to pawn her wedding ring, shawl and spare frocks to feed his insatiable addiction. She wrote in her diary of 'this damned Baden, this foul little town where we have been so unhappy'. He finally kicked the gambling habit in 1871 in Wiesbaden, where it had started nine years earlier. He was helped to quit by the continuing ministrations of the Orthodox priest, Father Yarishev, and also by Anna's resolve in refusing to send him 30 thalers which he promised he would return to her, but she well knew he would gamble away. It probably also helped that the following year the new German kaiser banned gambling across the entire German Empire. Dostoyevsky returned to a German *Kurort* four times before his death in 1881, going to Bad Ems to take the waters for his increasingly serious respiratory problems. On the whole, he felt that his cures there were effective, although drinking from the Kesselbrunnen spring gave him alternating constipation and diarrhoea. In other respects he had little good to say about the place. The wine was expensive vinegar, the shopkeepers were rude and charged exorbitant prices and the bands played nothing but Lutheran hymns and Wagner, whom he regarded as 'a most dull German dog in spite of his fame'.

Dostoyevsky was not the only mid-nineteenth-century writer to make gambling in a spa casino the major theme for a novel. Indeed, when novels of this period featured spas it was almost always the gambling that they majored on. It is a key theme in Frances Trollope's 1848 novel *The Robertses on Their Travels* and Edmond About's 1859 novel *Trente et Quarante*, both set in Baden-Baden. When About's novel was translated into English, it was given the title *Rouge et Noir: A Tale of Baden-Baden*. Rouge et Noir was a card game, also known as Trente et Quarante, which was hugely popular before it was supplanted by roulette in German *Kurorte* around 1850. In Anthony Trollope's *Can You Forgive Her?* (1865) gambling in the casino at Baden-Baden causes tensions between Plantagenet Palliser and his wife, Lady Glencora. While walking through the gaming room at the Assembly House makes him wish he had stayed in London, she finds herself seduced by its atmosphere and indeed by the whole hedonistic character of the spa, as she tells her companion, Alice Vavasor:

> I'll tell you what I want – something to live for – some excitement. Is it not a shame that I see around me so many people getting amusement, and that I can get none? I'd go and sit out there, and drink beer and hear the music, only Plantagenet wouldn't let me. I think I'll throw one piece onto the table to see what becomes of it.

To the horror of the prudish Alice, who tells her that while the croupiers raking in the money appear bad enough, the women betting on a card game round the table 'look like fiends', Lady

Glencora puts a gold Napoleon coin on one of the marked compartments. Three times she wins substantial amounts, always betting all her winnings on the next game. On the fourth try she loses everything just as her husband arrives furious 'that I find my wife playing at a common gambling table, surrounded by all that is wretched and vile – established there, seated, with heaps of gold before her' (Trollope 1989: 625–9).

Gambling and flirting quite often combine in the novels set in spa casinos. William Thackeray's 1850 Christmas story *The Kickleburys on the Rhine* features the fictional *Kurort* of Rougetnoirbourg, based on Bad Homburg, where 'the King of Trumps now virtually reigns' and 'there were women whose husbands, and men whose wives were left at home'. As Violet Hunt noted in her 1913 travelogue, *The Desirable Alien*, Thackeray 'cast around German thermal springs that vague aroma of *dévergondage*, that intimate flavour of impropriety, of possible scabrous adventure which appeals so deeply and intimately to the middle-class for which he catered' (Hunt 1913: 96). The opening passage of George Eliot's *Daniel Deronda* (1876), yet another novel set in Baden-Baden, finds the eponymous hero occupied in gambling 'in one of those splendid resorts which the enlightenment of ages has prepared for the same species of pleasure at a heavy cost of gilt mouldings, dark-toned colour and chubby nudities'. Eliot paints a picture of the 'very distant varieties of European type' assembled round the two long gaming tables as 'a striking admission of human equality'. In close proximity are an English countess, a raddled and withered old crone, a respectable London tradesman, a handsome Italian and a 'man with the air of an emaciated beau or worn-out libertine'. While every player differs markedly from every other, 'there was a certain uniform negativeness of expression which had the effect of a mask – as if they had all eaten of some root that for the time compelled the brains of each to the same narrow monotony of action.' Deronda finds his eyes drawn to a sylph-like young lady who is on a winning streak. His gaze seems to act as an evil eye and she starts losing until she has lost her 'last poor heap of napoleons'. They look at each other and so begins his doomed love affair with Gwendolen Harleth (Eliot 1984: 3–7).

There is a similar inter-mingling of gambling with what will ultimately be another hopelessly doomed love affair in Henry James's 1874 short story, 'Eugene Pickering'. The setting here is Bad Homburg and the atmosphere is perfectly evoked in the opening paragraph:

> The evening was very warm, and all the world was gathered on the terrace of the Kursaal, and the esplanade below it, to listen to the excellent orchestra; or half the world, rather, for the crowd was equally dense in the gaming-rooms, around the tables. The night was perfect, the season was at its height, the open windows of the Kursaal sent long shafts of unnatural light into the dusky woods, and now and then, in the intervals of the music, one might almost hear the clink of the napoleons and the metallic call of the croupiers rise above the watching silence of the saloons.

The unnamed narrator, sitting on one of the few vacant chairs, is drawn to a young man and a 'wonderfully pretty' middle-aged lady dressed in white muslin who is trying to catch his eye. Although at Homburg, 'one could never be sure', it does not appear that she is a courtesan, one of those 'whose especial vocation it was to catch a gentleman's eye'. Eventually, 'raising an ungloved hand, covered altogether with blue-gemmed rings – turquoises, sapphires and lapis – she beckoned him to come to her'. Self-conscious and blushing, he makes his way towards her. She asks him to play for her and soon in some embarrassment he is laying a coin on the table. Momentarily diverted by having to make way for 'a lady with a great many flounces', when the narrator looks again at the lady in white muslin, 'she was drawing in a very goodly pile of gold with her little blue-gemmed claw.' So begins an intense but ultimately doomed romance between the young Eugene Pickering, engaged to a woman he does not love, and the widowed Madame Blumenthal, played out in the steamy atmosphere of the spa casino and assembly rooms (James 1999: 36–41).

Another of Henry James's short stories, 'Confidence', published in 1880 and set in Baden-Baden, also mixes gambling and love-making. Catching perfectly the elegant mask and veneer that so often concealed the seedy reality of spa life, he describes the casino as 'the great temple of hazard, of as chaste an architecture as if it had been devoted to a much purer divinity' (James 1921: 20). The amatory atmosphere is made very clear in the letter that the hero Gordon Wright, an American scientist, sends to a friend after a few months in the *Kurort*: 'Do you know what I am doing? I am making love ... I have been making love ever since the last of May' (James 1921: 15).

There is generally more about gambling than there is about flirting and considerably more about both these activities than about the waters in the many nineteenth-century novels set in spas, and this is also true of much travel writing and even of several guidebooks. Henry James noted that describing Bad Homburg without mentioning gambling would be like 'writing about *Hamlet* with Hamlet himself omitted'. An 1858 guidebook to *The Beauties of Baden-Baden* took a similar line: 'It is well known that if you take away the gaming tables, you take away the attraction.' Bad Homburg's promotion of its 'magnificent casino' provoked an article in *Punch* in the same year taking a more censorious line. Noting that 'it requires some immoral courage to advertise a gambling house', it commented that the directors of the spa might as well go on to say that 'Homburg affords, in the gambling department, a supplement to the waters, enabling all parties to get themselves completely cleaned out' (*Punch* 1858: 105). Warnings abounded about the dangers of gambling and the sharp practices found in the casinos of German *Kurorte*. As early as 1826 Benjamin Disraeli's novel *Vivian Grey* featured a 'vile conspiracy' involving marked cards at Bad Ems. The Russian journalist Nikolai Grech warned in 1843 that in Baden-Baden 'it very often happens that gamblers have their purses swiped from their pockets' (Grech 1843: 209). In England there were periodic moralistic outbursts about the iniquities of women gambling. Echoing the outrage of Plantagenet Palliser, an Anglican clergyman, Joel Headley, found himself overcome with feelings of revulsion when he saw a beautiful and clearly upper-class lady sitting with 'her delicate white hand on a pile of money' at the gaming table in Baden-Baden on a visit in 1845: 'I did not think it was possible for an elegant and well-dressed young lady to fill me with feelings of such utter disgust. Her very beauty became ugliness and her auburn tresses looked more unbecoming than the elfin locks of a sorceress' (Headley 1845: 104). In 1862 a correspondent to *St James's Magazine* warned that respectable women taking an evening walk behind the casino in Wiesbaden were likely to be taken for prostitutes.

Despite the warnings, women as well as men continued flocking in ever greater numbers to the gaming rooms in the Continental spas. Russians were the most enthusiastic gamblers, as Dostoyevsky and Tolstoy testified by their behaviour as well as their writings. Among the most prodigious was the Countess Sophie Kissileff, who spent virtually every day from 11 a.m. to 11 p.m. in the casino at Bad Homburg during the season throughout the 1850s. She is said to have lost the equivalent of over four million dollars (more than £3.2 million) in today's money. According to some accounts, she owned shares in the casino so perhaps some of what she lost at least came back in the form of dividends. The Russian writer Mikhail Lermontov identified among his compatriots 'a class apart amongst those who place their hopes in the medicinal waters: They drink – but not water – take but few walks, indulge in only mild flirtations, but gamble, and complain of boredom' (Lermontov 1912: 169).

Russians were not immune to the other more common form of *Kurschatten* and enjoyed the pleasures of flirting in spas. An 1815 play, *A School for Coquettes*, set at the Lipetsk springs, was the first in a series of Russian works of fiction featuring spas as places of sexual adventure and healing. *Erotida*, a novel written in 1835 by Aleksandr Veltman, describes a group of testosterone-charged Russian soldiers in the Napoleonic Wars heading for a spa during a brief period of leave seeking 'water and love at 165 degrees' (Morgan 2014: 87). A cartoon in a Moscow newspaper in 1873 featured two elderly ladies, one asking 'And what effect did Vichy have on you?', and the other, a matchmaker, replying 'Outstanding! Prince Andrei has begun to court Zina.'

In flirting, as in gambling, Baden-Baden's reputation was second to none. Among those who experienced *Kurschatten* there were a trio of well-known composers. Franz Liszt brought his mistress, the wild Irish dancer and singer, Lola Montez, in 1845. She frequented the roulette tables, on one occasion throwing a leg over the shoulder of the man standing next to her, distracting both the gamblers and the croupier, and on another raising her skirt so high to impress an admirer in the Konversationshaus that she was expelled from the town. Hector Berlioz came ten times to conduct the resident orchestra at the invitation of Edouard Bénazet, and his *Béatrice et Bénédict* was the opening production at the new theatre in 1862. One of the attractions of his regular visits was the chance to treat his severe nervous disorder, diagnosed as 'intestinal neuralgia', which caused him acute pain. His *Kurschatten* experience seems to have been brief and unhappy, as described by his friend Ernest Legouvé, who reported meeting the composer in the woods below the old castle on the outskirts of the town: 'He seemed different, aged and sad. We sat on a bench, for the climb tired him. He was holding a letter, which he clutched convulsively. It was from a young and pretty girl in love with him but he said regretfully: "I am nearly sixty. She cannot love me – she does not love me" '(Bradley 2010: 92). Johannes Brahms spent every summer in Baden-Baden between 1864 and 1872, coming there principally because of his attraction to Clara Schumann, who had taken up residence in the Lichtentaler Allee with her seven children at the suggestion of her old friend Pauline Viardot-García, following the death of her husband. Brahms became infatuated with Clara's twenty-two-year-old daughter Julie. In 1869, hearing from Clara that Julie had accepted a proposal of marriage from an Italian count, a distraught Brahms poured his grief and loneliness into the *Alto Rhapsody* (Opus 53), a setting of a poem by Goethe. A week after attending Julie's wedding he turned up at Clara's house and played the piece to her. She wrote in her journal 'It is long since I remember being so moved by a depth of pain in words and music … This piece seems to me neither more nor less than an expression of his own heart's anguish' (Swafford 1998: 351).

The outbreak of the Franco-Prussian War in 1870 had a major impact on Baden-Baden. The French stopped coming and the liberal cosmopolitan atmosphere disappeared in the face of a much more authoritarian and puritanical political climate. The banning of gambling in the new German Empire led to the closure of the casino at the end of the 1872 season and heralded the end of the spa's reign as the summer resort of Europe's playboys. The number of *Kurgäste* halved in 1873, an indication of just how many had come there primarily to gamble. The casino remained closed until 1933 when the Nazis reopened it to raise hard cash. Other German *Kurorte* suffered a similar decline. The number of *Kurgäste* in Bad Ems fell by a third through the 1870s and its casino was not reopened until 1987. Gambling was also banned in Belgium in 1872. To compensate for the loss of revenue from the casino, the town of Spa received 890,000 francs (around €4.5 million or £3.6 million today) from the government which was spent on building the Galerie Leopold II and the Protestant and Catholic churches.

Mark Twain visited Baden-Baden eight years after the outbreak of the Franco-Prussian War as part of his 'tramp' around Europe. Like so many other visitors, he took a rather jaundiced view of the place, acknowledging the beauty of its setting, parks and buildings, but describing it as 'an inane town, filled with sham, and petty fraud, and snobbery'. He did, however, concede that 'the baths are good. I spoke with many people, and they were all agreed in that.' Twain initially felt that the large numbers of people 'who march back and forth past the music stand and look very much bored' made the lot of the *Kurgast* 'a rather aimless and stupid existence' but he subsequently tempered his view, reflecting that 'a good many of these people are there for a real purpose; they are racked with rheumatism, and they are there to stew it out in the hot baths.' Although he did not find their appearance very encouraging – 'these invalids looked melancholy enough, limping about on their canes and crutches, and apparently brooding over all sorts of cheerless things' – he conceded that the baths seemed effective, not least in his own case. After a fortnight's bathing there, the rheumatism that he had suffered unceasingly for three years had departed:

> I fully believe I left my rheumatism in Baden-Baden. Baden-Baden is welcome to it. It was little, but it was all I had to give. I would have preferred to leave something that was catching, but it was not in my power. (Twain 1996: 200)

In his notes on Baden-Baden, Twain focused largely on the waters, giving detailed descriptions of the experience of taking a bath in the new Friedrichsbad in a large marble bath tub full of water at a temperature of 35 degrees Celsius (95 degrees Fahrenheit) and of drinking in the *Trinkhalle* his prescribed doses of the hot water 'with a spoonful of salt from the Carlsbad springs dissolved in it. That is not a dose to be forgotten right away.' He wrote nothing about gambling or womanising, although he did complain about the mercenary spirit of the local traders and their keenness to extract every last penny out of the hapless *Kurgäste*.

Other foreign visitors coming to Baden-Baden around this time felt that it had become altogether too pleased with itself and lost its original therapeutic purpose in becoming simply a playground for the idle rich, full of shallow poseurs and charlatans. The Russian writer Mikhail Saltykov-Shchedrin commented during a stay in 1867: 'I encountered an entire troupe of people who revelled in their own idleness, stupidity and swagger ... I had never in my life seen such a perfect group of fops' (Morgan 2014: 265). An American journalist visiting Saratoga Springs in 1868 had a similar reaction: 'Never, in the whole course of my life, had I seen such manifest signs of the general possession of wealth accompanied by such a widespread lack of refinement ... Once Saratoga was a whited sepulchre; now, it is a sepulchre without any whitewash whatever. The *crème de la crème* is a bad quality of skimmed milk, and Saratoga is a huge cauldron, bubbling over with vice and frivolity' (Chambers 2002: 215). On both sides of the Atlantic, it seemed to many observers that spas had become decadent empty shells, their former glories dissipated in an orgy of hedonism and conspicuous consumption.

It was partly in reaction to these trends that a new much simpler and more austere type of water-based cure was emerging and gaining popularity. It challenged the decadence and the elegance of Europe's traditional spas but it did not totally efface them. They were to have a final glorious flourishing in the closing decades of the nineteenth century and the opening decade of the twentieth, that period known as La Belle Époque, when Baden-Baden's mantle passed to Karlsbad and Marienbad. Before chronicling that episode in the history of spas, we need to turn away from *der Kurschatten* and the lure of the roulette table, take a short, sharp shower of cold water, wrap up in wet sheets, get plenty of exercise in the fresh air and adopt a Spartan diet. Such were the vigorous, bracing, no-nonsense elements at the heart of the hydrotherapy movement which gained numerous adherents on both sides of the Atlantic in the second half of the nineteenth century.

6

HYDROTHERAPY – A SHORT SHARP DOUCHE OF COLD WATER

The leading European spas had built their reputation on the basis of the chemical composition and therapeutic properties of their naturally mineral-rich and sometimes also naturally heated waters, and the many attractions which they offered to those resorting to them to take the cure. In the mid-nineteenth century a new, simpler but more demanding kind of water-based cure arose that did not depend on any special mineral properties in the water and did not countenance any diversions, certainly not gambling or flirting. All that was needed was ordinary tap water, and a strict regime involving lots of fresh air, a plain wholesome diet washed down with copious draughts of water and not much else, hours wrapped in wet towels and frequent cold showers and douches.

The two pioneers of this new science of hydrotherapy were Vincent Priessnitz, a peasant farmer from Silesia, and Sebastian Kneipp, a Catholic priest from Bavaria. Both men were deeply religious and their approach, which focused firmly on health and shunned any kind of hedonism, appealed to high-minded Victorians uneasy about the growing frivolity and decadence of spas. Their techniques were widely taken up, not least in Britain and the United States, and hydrotherapy became one of the most popular forms of alternative medicine in the nineteenth century, eclipsing both homeopathy and hypnosis.

The benefits to health of drinking and bathing in ordinary cold water, which had been recognised in ancient times by the likes of

Hippocrates and Galen, were vigorously championed by a number of doctors and other enthusiasts in the eighteenth century. In 1702 John Floyer, a doctor in Lichfield, published an essay on the merits of cold bathing, which was to have considerably more influence on the Continent than in his native England. Four years later another English physician, Edward Baynard, suggested that bathing in cold river water conferred just as much benefit as immersion in Bath's thermal mineral waters. He cited the case of 'a certain Archdeacon, who when he was a student at Oxford, eating too much fat venison, found himself extremely ill.' He plunged into the Thames 'and swam up and down for the space of near two hours, and came forth very well and continued so' (Lennard 1931: 74–5). Across Europe, societies were set up to promote the medicinal use of water. Among the most extreme was the Société Acquavite set up in Geneva in 1714 by a British soldier, Lieutenant Cordier, who left the army to follow a severely ascetic lifestyle. Believing that it was 'the vital force' of life, he and his followers lived off copious draughts of water and not much else. He later advocated living on nothing but air and died through putting this theory into practice.

John Wesley, the Anglican clergyman remembered as the founder of Methodism, was a prominent advocate of water as an aid to health. His *Primitive Physic*, published in 1747, extolled the benefits of both drinking and bathing in it alongside other components of a healthy lifestyle such as fresh air, exercise and good plain food. 'Drink only water, if it agrees with your stomach,' he wrote, 'if not, good, clear small beer.' Spirituous liquors should be avoided, along with coffee and tea, especially for those with weak nerves. He recommended that everyone should have a cold bath on rising in the morning:

> Cold bathing is of great advantage to health: it prevents abundance of diseases. It promotes perspiration, helps the circulation of the blood, and prevents the danger of catching cold. Tender people should pour water upon the head before they go in, and walk in swiftly. (Wesley 1858: ix)

Wesley offered more specific prescriptions for both bathing in and drinking water in the case of particular conditions. He recommended pregnant women to take cold baths two or three times a week to avoid miscarriage and those suffering from chronic headaches to bathe their feet in warm water for a quarter of an hour before going to bed. Cold baths were prescribed as the main cure for more than fifty afflictions, including ague, apoplexy, asthma, burns, cholic, convulsions, corns, dropsy, falling sickness, leprosy, palsy, rheumatism, rickets, sciatica and involuntary urinating. Consumptives were advised to drink nothing but spring water and those with a cold or a fever to drink a pint to a pint and a half of cold water while lying down in bed. He cited the case of a woman who had suffered from breast cancer for thirteen years and been cured by a mixture of daily cold baths for a month, drinking only water and applying red poppy water and rose water, mixed with honey and roses, to the affected area.

By the late eighteenth century a growing number of doctors across Europe were enthusiastically throwing pails of water over their patients in the belief that this was doing them good. It was in the German-speaking world that a more formalised and systematic approach to curing through water developed in the early nineteenth century with the emergence of hydrotherapy, also known as hydropathy, based on the repeated action of water as an agent, either applied externally to the body or taken internally. The man generally taken to be its founding father, Vincent Priessnitz (1799–1851), was the son of a peasant farmer in the tiny hamlet of Graefenberg in the remote mountainous region of Silesia on the northern edge of the Austro-Hungarian Empire. The village is now known as Jeseník and is in the north-east part of the Czech Republic near the Polish border. As a young boy Priessnitz would often rest beneath the shade of a tree close to a spring. He watched a young roe deer which had been shot in the thigh drag itself to the spring and submerge its wounded limb in flowing water. Over a period of several days he observed the animal return again and again to the spring and gradually regain its strength.

This experience left the young Priessnitz with a strong sense of both the spiritual power and the healing properties of water. By the age of fifteen he had become the unofficial medical adviser to his village, recommending people to use cold water to treat their bruises and injuries. After a serious accident when he was run over by a wagon laden with oats, he managed to cure himself by strapping cold wet bandages across his chest and drinking copious quantities of cold water to prevent fever. He went on wearing the bandages for a year. The application of similar compresses, known as 'dripping sheets', was at the heart of the hydrotherapy that he started to practise professionally in 1819. He extended his water cure from just treating sprains and surface injuries by developing what he called the 'sweat cure' for chronic illnesses. This involved encouraging patients to sweat in bed and then immersing them in tubs full of cold water, pouring buckets of water over their heads and rubbing their skin. Altogether, he developed fifty-six varieties of water-based treatments from foot compresses and wet sheets to powerful douches. His fame became such that people started coming to Graefenberg from far afield and in 1822 he rebuilt his home to be the first dedicated hydropathic establishment in the world. At the heart of his philosophy, expounded in several books which became bestsellers, was a call to a serious and single-minded dedication to the water cure, very different from the half-hearted commitment expected of those who frequented spas. He forbade his patients from discussing their illnesses, insisted that they show total devotion to the recovery of their health, 'not living partly as patients and partly in search of pleasure', and warned that 'those who have a weak character, or show no inclination to strengthen it, had better remain away from the water cure' (Metcalfe 1898: 86).

Priessnitz received powerful official endorsement in 1838 when an Imperial Commission appointed to investigate his hydropathic establishment gave it a glowing report and recommended that he

be granted similar privileges to members of the medical profession
and given a licence to practise. Among his many well-connected
patients were the Habsburg Archduke Franz Karl and the prince-
bishop of Breslau. The number of visitors coming to Graefenberg
to take the water cure rose from fifty-four in 1830 to 1,700, of
whom 120 were themselves doctors, in 1839. Alongside cold
baths, showers and wet sheet packs, his cure involved drinking
large quantities of cold water – he recommended ten to twelve
glasses a day – abstinence from alcohol, a simple diet and lots of
fresh air and exercise. There were no distractions, as this account
by a patient testifies:

> Up in the early morning, often before 5 am, sweating through dry
> compresses followed by a full cold bath. Then breakfast, spartanly
> simple with black bread, butter and cold milk. One or two hours
> after breakfast, a climb up the Graefenberg, a walk of some thirty
> minutes. Once up, remove all clothes, whatever the weather,
> and shower in ice-cold mountain spring water which had been
> harnessed and streamed from different heights. At midday, a meal
> together; broth, pudding, fruit and salad. From 3.30 pm repeat
> the morning cure. 7 pm, supper as breakfast. Bed. (Hahn 1980:
> 94)

A number of Priessnitz's grateful patients erected elaborate
monuments and fountains dedicated to him which can still be seen
on the wooded hills around Jeseník. He also acquired a growing
band of disciples among doctors. Within forty years of his death,
over 400 books had been written about the 'water doctor', as he
was hailed, and numerous hydropathic establishments had been set
up across Europe, not least in Britain. One of his most enthusiastic
British disciples, Richard Claridge, an asphalt contractor and militia
captain, returned home after a three-month stay at Graefenberg in
1841 completely cured of his chronic rheumatism, having taken,
on his careful calculation, 800 cold baths, drunk 1,500 tumblers of

water, walked 1,000 miles and perspired for 200 hours. He devoted much of the rest of his life to touring the British Isles attempting to persuade his compatriots of the benefits of the water cure which he also promoted in his bestselling book *Hydropathy; or The Cold Water Cure, as practiced by Vincent Priessnitz* in which he noted rather despondently: 'The Germans drink a great deal of water, but the English carry their distaste for it so far, that many persons never drink half a pint of it, undiluted, at one time, in their lives' (Claridge 1843: 41).

Another of Priessnitz's satisfied patients was an English doctor who had become disillusioned with drug-based medicine, which he felt did more harm than good. In 1842 James Wilson came away from an eight-month stay at Graefenberg, where he calculated that he had drunk 3,500 tumblers of water and spent 480 hours in cold wet sheets, determined to set up a similar hydropathic establishment in England. He settled on Malvern in Worcestershire where the exceptionally pure water emerging from springs on the slopes of its famous hills already had a reputation for its curative properties. Indeed, what were effectively hydropathic treatments, although the word was not used, had been pursued there from the early 1800s, with a regime of bathing, drinking, early rising, exercise and temperance in all things prescribed for a range of ailments. Here, in contrast to spas, the water contained no mineral elements – indeed its efficacy, according to an eighteenth-century medical practitioner, rested on the fact that 'it contained just nothing at all.' Wilson bought the lease of an old hotel and turned it into Graefenberg House with rooms for ten to twelve patients. In 1845 he opened a much larger hydropathic establishment called Priessnitz House with accommodation for sixty patients.

Wilson was joined in Malvern by Dr James Gully who in 1846 wrote an influential manifesto, *The Water Cure in Chronic Disease,* which helped to establish hydropathy in Britain. Their success encouraged other 'water doctors' to set up practices and residential cure houses in the town. At the heart of the treatment they offered was the application of what was called 'the pack', which involved patients being wrapped from head to toe in wet sheets and then covered in blankets, leading to extensive perspiration. Priessnitz had emphasised the importance of inducing a 'crisis' which produced fever, skin eruptions and boils to drive poisons out of the system. John Leech, a contributor to *Punch*, described the cure which he took in 1850 in *Three Weeks in Wet Sheets, being the Diary and Doings of a Moist Visitor to Malvern*. It provides a chilling description of the daily regime for patients which began with being wrapped tightly in cold wet sheets at 5 a.m. and smothered in blankets for an hour, followed by a sitz or sitting bath while cold water was poured over the head either from watering cans or from a cistern-like contraption which released 150 gallons in a continuous stream. Next came a brisk walk to one of the springs in the Malvern Hills, from which patients were expected to drink up to eighteen tumblers. Only after these rigours were complete was a meagre ration of porridge, milk, toast and weak cold tea provided for breakfast. The rest of the day was occupied by more treatments, including the application for many hours of an abdominal compress consisting of a tightly bound sheet regularly soaked in cold water, visits to the countryside and improving lectures, alleviated only by lunch of boiled mutton and rice pudding, an early evening 'hydropathic tea' of white bread, butter and treacle washed down with more water, followed by an early bed. Variations on this standard treatment included a lamp bath, where the patient sat swathed in wet blankets over a heated paraffin lamp to induce perspiration and replicate the effect of a Turkish bath, and a compressed air bath, which increased the atmospheric pressure and was said to be good for asthma. Leech commented that:

> Anybody you meet, like yourself, is steaming with moisture –
> however gorgeously the old Dowager is dressed, at night she's
> in reality underneath as moist as a frog. The fair young beauty is
> but a water lily up to her armpits in that element and the curry-
> eating old Indian is hissing like an urn-iron in a suit full of wet
> swaddling clothes. (Harcup 2010: 38)

This moist atmosphere was compounded by an ethos akin to monasticism and muscular Christianity in the Malvern hydropathic establishments where the minimum stay was a fortnight, although a month was regarded as preferable. Dr Wilson imposed a severe regime, going round on his horse whipping those who dawdled on their morning walk up the steep Malvern Hills. Believing that a water cure offered the best remedy for 'the evils of a stomach generally overworked, and a skin under-worked', he set an example to his patients by regularly consuming up to thirty flasks of water before breakfast, pointing out 'you wash your face with water, so why not your stomach too?' Alcohol, smoking and sugary treats were absolutely forbidden to patients. The puritanical atmosphere is well described in a book published in 1845 entitled *Confessions of a Water Patient* by Edward Bulwer-Lytton, the politician and poet responsible for coining the phrase 'the great unwashed', who spent ten weeks taking a cure in Malvern. On one occasion he was discovered by Wilson in the town with a bag of tarts concealed under his coat. He claimed that he had bought them for a lady friend, eliciting Wilson's response: 'Poison! Throw them down in the gutter at once, and have more respect for her insides.' Bulwer-Lytton also records the hasty departure of a female patient who was expelled because 'the doctor has found tarts, and other improprieties, concealed in her drawers' (Harcup 2010: 47).

Several eminent Victorians subjected themselves to the water cure. Alfred Tennyson, who suffered throughout his life from a pervasive melancholy and depression, diagnosed in the fashion of the times as gout, took his first hydropathic treatment in 1844, at a time when his son Hallam noted that 'so severe a hypochondria set in upon him that his friends despaired of his life.' He spent seven months at an establishment near Cheltenham which he described as 'the only one in England conducted on pure Priessnitzian principles' – it was run by Priessnitz's nephew – and enthusiastically reported that he had experienced 'four crises (one larger than had been seen for two or three years in Graefenberg, indeed I believe the largest but one that has been seen) and much poison has come out of me which no physic ever would have brought to light' (Tennyson 1982: 222). His brother, Horatio, who undertook a cure there at the same time, was less enthusiastic, noting that it 'chiefly consists of a series of packings and unpackings. You are packed in a wet sheet two or three times a day and each time on coming out you are plunged into a cold bath after which you have a wet bandage tightly bound around your waist, you are also occasionally thawed and dissolved into a dew by being swathed in three or four blankets on the removal of which, greatly to your disgust you are again plunged into stinging cold water' (Martin 1980: 277). Alfred Tennyson went to Malvern in 1847 and 1848 as a patient of Dr Gully, who told him that much of his recurrent ill health was attributable to his habit of consuming a bottle of port daily. On his discharge, he was under orders to have no more than two glasses a day and also to quit smoking, commandments that he failed to keep. Following his various hydropathic treatments, he seems to have shaken off the 'hypochondria' which had led him to try the water cure although he did have a five-week stay in Harrogate in 1863 to drink the waters there.

Charles Darwin, who had lifelong bouts of abdominal pain, flatulence and headaches which modern biographers have tended to attribute either to hypochondria or to a tropical disease inflicted by insect bites on his travels in South America, was persuaded to try treatment at Dr Gully's hydropathic establishment in 1849 following four months of incessant vomiting. Gully agreed with Darwin's self-diagnosis of nervous dyspepsia and prescribed the usual mixture of packing with sheets, cold baths, wearing a wet compress all day, long walks and a strict diet. Although his sixteen-week stay induced 'the most complete stagnation of mind', Darwin's health improved considerably, and he concluded that the water cure was 'no quackery'. After returning home, he continued with the diet and set up a special shed in his garden with apparatus to administer cold showers. He returned to Malvern for a further cure in 1850 and when his ten-year-old daughter Annie suffered persistent nausea and weight loss the following year, he took her to be treated by Dr Gully. Despite repeated assurances that she was recovering, she died from bilious fever after a few weeks. Darwin was heartbroken at her death, which weakened his Christian faith and prompted reflection about extermination of the weak through natural selection and evolution. Annie's grave can still be seen in the grounds of Malvern Priory.

Thomas Carlyle took himself to Malvern in 1851 in an effort to cure chronic stomach and bowel problems. Dr Gully seems to have succeeded in convincing him that his problems were more in the mind than in the body but Carlyle was not enthusiastic about his experience, noting that he had found 'water, taken as a medicine, to be the most destructive drug I had ever tried' (Martin 1980: 277). Charles Dickens, who accompanied his wife for a stay in the same year, complained at Dr Wilson's prohibition of snuff, 'that chief solace in life', and wrote a one-act play set in the fictional Water-Lily Hotel in Malvern where a Mr Gabblewig came to discover if the cold-water cure could repair his broken heart.

Florence Nightingale was almost certainly Malvern's most regular eminent patient. She first came for a course of hydrotherapy in 1857 when she was exhausted by her harrowing nursing work in the Crimean War, a victim of what would now be called post-traumatic stress disorder, and also suffering from brucellosis. She returned for at least eight more cures over the next twelve years and although her condition left her through much of this period an invalid confined to a couch or chair in her room, she reckoned that her hydropathic treatments added three years to her life. Like many spa patients, she found that her lengthy cures induced a sense of isolation and introspection. When her father visited her, he found her sitting alone in the top room of the hydropathic house staring out of the window: 'There was a sort of solemn isolation from an outward world. She sat alone looking over the great plain, meditating from her window like one of her own Prophets looking towards Jerusalem' (Harcup 2010: 81). Her diary entries during her stays in Malvern indicate that she observed among her fellow patients the mixture of hypochondria and valetudinarianism so commonly found in spa guests:

> Hydropathy has become a highly popular amusement among athletic individuals, who have felt the *tedium vitae* and those indefinite diseases which a large income and unbounded leisure are so well calculated to produce. (Harcup 2010: 80)

Drs Wilson and Gully parted company after a few years and both came to rather sad ends. Wilson died of a heart attack in 1867 while preparing to enter a tepid bath in a hydropathic establishment in Yorkshire where he had gone to seek relief from the dyspepsia which had first taken him to Graefenberg. Gully had his own *Kurschatten* experience, falling for a young married woman, Florence Ricardo, who consulted him about her depression in 1870. Her alcoholic husband, whom she had persuaded to seek treatment from him, died suddenly in Cologne the following year and in 1872 Gully, recently retired from his Malvern practice, took off with Florence to Bad Kissingen. On their return, she found that she was pregnant and Gully performed a secret abortion. Florence subsequently met and fell in love with Charles Bravo, whom she married in 1875, provoking Gully into a fit of jealous rage. Just a few months later Bravo died of poisoning. The poison was traced to Malvern, where it had been bought to treat Gully's horses, and he was suspected of the murder although his involvement was never proved. Despite these setbacks, Malvern continued as Britain's leading hydropathic centre. By 1870 it had three hydropathic establishments and 300 lodging houses. Treatments supervised by the town's numerous 'water doctors' continued well into the twentieth century.

It was not only doctors who set up hydropathic establishments in Britain. John Smedley, a Derbyshire hosiery manufacturer and ardent Methodist who had been cured of enteric fever through hydropathy, established one at Matlock in 1853. He offered an extensive menu of 223 bath treatments, headed by the Cold Dripping Sheet, and imposed a stern regime on patients, beginning and ending the day with worship, banning alcohol and tobacco and punishing those who arrived late for meals. Holding conventional doctors and clergy of the established church in equal contempt, Smedley's enthusiasm for hydropathy was informed by his fervent Nonconformist evangelicalism. He likened the water cure to the experience of becoming a born-again Christian.

It was probably its clean-living, disciplined, puritanical ethos that led the hydropathic movement to be taken up with particular alacrity in Presbyterian Scotland. The first Scottish hydro, as they became known, was set up in 1843 in Rothesay on the Isle of Bute with a further twenty being established over the next forty years. Most were run by strongly evangelical Christians, like Dr Thomas Meikle, founder of the Strathearn (later Crieff) Hydropathic in 1848, who was a devout member of the United Presbyterian Church and a temperance reformer. He had Pindar's motto 'Water is Best' inlaid in the floor of the entrance hall and instituted the practice, which persisted well into the twentieth century, of serving every guest with a glass of hot water just before bedtime, which like other fixed points in the day was rigidly prescribed and signalled by the ringing of a bell. The Scottish hydros were run on strict religious principles, with grace before meals, morning and evening prayers, full Sunday services and a ban on alcoholic refreshment. They became favourite resorts of respectable middle-class, church-going families although some found their religious atmosphere rather off-putting. Noting that fines were imposed on those who arrived for meals after grace had been said or those who discussed details of their treatments, an American guest at Crieff Hydro in 1904 wrote: 'We cannot decide whether we are in a boarding school or theological training house' (Bradley 2012: 170).

It was a Scotsman who became the chief promoter of another nineteenth-century fad closely associated with hydrotherapy, although in this case involving hot rather than cold water. David Urquhart, a diplomat and MP, developed an obsession with the benefits of Turkish baths which he had encountered during his time at the British Embassy in Constantinople in the 1830s. He was instrumental in introducing Turkish baths into Britain in the 1850s and 1860s and wrote a somewhat eccentric pamphlet suggesting that their widespread introduction in Ireland would solve the social and political problems in that part of the United Kingdom. He argued that the Irish peasantry were despised by the Anglo-Irish aristocracy as 'the great unwashed'. Installing a Turkish bath in every village would make them cleaner than their social betters, who 'misguidedly soaked themselves in tubfuls of their own dirty water', and so end the animosity and oppression which was at the root of the vexed Irish question. Urquhart's unusual proposal for solving the Irish question was never put into practice, although Turkish baths, with their hallmark Moorish-style tiles and arches, were built in many British towns and cities in the later nineteenth century.

The water cure as established by Priessnitz remained popular in its German-speaking homeland. Among those who regularly submitted himself to its rigours was Richard Wagner. Like many other nineteenth-century composers, he regularly visited spas, notably Teplitz, Karlsbad and Marienbad. He was not a natural spa patient, however. During one bathing session in Marienbad in 1845 he felt an overpowering desire to write out a new theme for his opera *Lohengrin* and jumped out of the water, which he was supposed to stay in for an hour, after a few minutes. His doctor told him that he had better give up taking spa cures as he was clearly quite unfit for them. Instead, he became a convert to hydrotherapy, attracted by 'its bold repudiation of the entire science of medicine, with all its quackeries, combined with its advocacy of the simplest natural processes' (Wagner 1911: 569). He credited an exclusive water regime based on Priessnitz's principles with curing him from the effects of sulphur baths, prescribed for a rash over his entire body, which had left him in a 'severe state of irritability'. In September 1851, feeling particularly dejected, he booked himself into a hydropathic establishment at Albisbrunnen about three miles from his home in Zürich:

> Early at five o'clock in the morning I was wrapped up and kept in a state of perspiration for several hours; after that I was plunged into an icy cold bath at a temperature of only four degrees; then I was made to take a brisk walk to restore my circulation in the chilly air of late autumn. In addition I was kept on a water diet; no wine, coffee, or tea was allowed; and this regime, in the dismal company of nothing but incurables, with dull evenings only enlivened by desperate attempts at games of whist, and the prohibition of all intellectual occupation, resulted in irritability and overwrought nerves. I led this life for nine weeks, but I was determined not to give in until I felt that every kind of drug or poison I had ever absorbed into my system had been brought to the surface. (Wagner 1911: 572–3)

During his lengthy cure, Wagner consoled himself by thinking of all the wine that he had imbibed over many evening dinner parties 'and which must evaporate in profuse perspiration'. He persuaded his friend, Karl Ritter, to come and join him in the treatment but Ritter proved an unsatisfactory patient, denouncing the use of cold milk as 'indigestible and against the dictates of Nature' and discovering 'a wretched confectioner's shop in the neighbouring village, where he was caught buying cheap pastry on the sly'.

Although he had periodic doubts about its efficacy, Wagner remained an enthusiast for hydrotherapy, the principles of which he adopted as 'a new kind of religion'. He fulminated against alcohol 'as an evil and barbarous substitute for the ecstatic state of mind which love alone should produce' and wrote that 'I continued on the coldest winter mornings to take my cold baths, and plagued my wife to death by making her show me the way out with a lantern for the prescribed early morning walk' (Wagner 1911: 622). In 1856, in an effort to gain relief from recurrent erysipelas (an unsightly and potentially dangerous skin infection), he checked into a hydropathic establishment near Geneva run by a doctor who had himself been cured of paralysis in both legs while under the care of Priessnitz. Wagner found his treatment, which lasted for two months and 'consisted in the most ingenious use of water at a moderate temperature', thoroughly calming and efficacious. During his absence his wife, Minna, took a sour-milk cure. Enthusiast though he was for hydrotherapy, Wagner did not subject himself to the rather alarming-sounding devices developed in the 1860s by a Viennese physician, Wilhelm Winternitz, to administer cold-water treatments which included rectum and vaginal coolers and a water-cooled catheter designed to tone the urinary tract.

Priessnitz's mantle passed in the later decades of the nineteenth century to Sebastian Kneipp (1821–97), who served from 1881 until his death as parish priest of the small village of Wörishofen in Bavaria where he achieved a similar reputation for his water-based cures. He, too, came to espouse hydrotherapy through direct personal experience, having apparently cured himself of pulmonary tuberculosis while a theological student by means of short immersions two or three times a week in the cold waters of the River Danube. Subsequently, he treated parishioners with a variety of complaints including cholera through a combination of wet wraps, cold baths, a strict vegetarian diet and regular exercise, including early-morning barefoot walks for forty-five minutes through the dewy grass. In 1891 he set up a special cure centre in Wörishofen for Catholic priests, the Sebastianeum, complete with elaborate neo-baroque chapel, and established his main consulting room there. His fame spread after he cured the Habsburg Archduke Joseph, commander-in-chief of the Hungarian army, from acute sciatica in 1892. The following year Pope Leo XIII made Kneipp a monsignor, much to the annoyance of the local apothecaries who had hoped he would receive a papal censure for ruining their business with his insistence on using natural remedies rather than drugs.

Kneipp's book *Meine Wasserkur* (*My Water Cure*), published in 1886 and translated into fourteen languages including English, made him an international celebrity. He toured Europe and many doctors came to Wörishofen to study his cure, which was based on five principles: hydrotherapy; kinesiotherapy (exercise and muscular movement through massage); phytotherapy (using medical plants and herbs); nutrition and diet; and what he described as '*Ordnung*', an ordered holistic lifestyle balancing body and soul. His championship of this particular combination of therapies has led his many devotees to hail him as the founding father of holistic medicine. Central to Kneipp's water cure was the application of affusions or '*Güsse*' of alternating hot and cold water on different parts of the body. Photographs show him standing in his cassock emptying the contents of watering cans over the backs of patients, or in one case directing a hose at the posterior of Baron de Bilguer. Like Priessnitz, Kneipp wrapped his patients in wet sheets and also got them to walk in cold-water baths and immerse their arms in special sinks. His insistence that female patients took off their shoes and stockings and hitched up their skirts to paddle in local streams and ponds led to Wörishofen being dubbed the 'sinful village' by outraged locals. By 1895 he was seeing nearly 2,000 patients a month.

Kneipp's regime was not as austere as that recommended by Priessnitz and practised in Malvern and the Scottish hydros. Although he advocated that the drink of choice 'should be the genuine beverage offered by God in every well', he went on to say, 'I am not a Puritan and allow gladly a glass of wine or beer, but without regarding them as important as they are commonly believed to be' (Kneipp 1894: 10). He himself drank alcohol and also often smoked a cigar. The corpulence evident in surviving photographs suggests that he did not stint himself in the 'dry, simple, nourishing household fare not spoiled by art or by strong spices' that he recommended to his patients.

Hydrotherapy became particularly popular in the United States. Around 200 hydropathic establishments were set up across the country in the 1840s and 1850s. As in Scotland, the movement had a strongly puritanical aspect. A tract published in 1844 on *Licentiousness and Its Effects Upon the Body and Mental Health* advocated 'the hydropathic management of masturbation', using the 'sweating process' to treat males guilty of the sin of onanism. This 'consisted of encouraging perspiration and then altering it with cold air and baths; in another method, a wet sheet was wrapped around the person and as soon as he became warm, the sheet was replaced with another' (Cayleff 1987: 55). Several prominent figures in American religious life were enthusiasts for hydrotherapy. Mary Baker Eddy, founder of the Church of Christ, Scientist, obtained relief from her chronic health problems through pursuing a course of treatment at a hydro in the mid-1850s. As a result of this experience, water became a key feature in the Christian Science programme of alternative medicine and along with fresh air, exercise and prayer, she recommended her followers to take a sip of pure water every half hour. Seventh-day Adventists also took up hydropathy. It was introduced at the Adventists' Health Reform Institute in Battle Creek, Michigan, by John Harvey Kellogg, the medical doctor and holistic health advocate best known as the inventor of cornflakes breakfast cereal, when he became superintendent there in 1874. Renamed the Battle Creek Sanitarium (sic), it was treating more than 7,000 patients by the end of the 1920s.

The United States' largest and most prestigious hydropathic establishment was set up in Saratoga Springs in the early 1930s as part of the New Deal to counter the effects of the Depression. It reinvigorated the medical side of this most European of all American spas which had looked in the 1920s as though it might completely lose its therapeutic purpose – a visiting journalist noted at the beginning of that decade that 'whilst an occasional invalid does come, he does not stay long; he moves too slowly and requires too much attention to be either welcome or benefited, and he is practically crowded out by the 999 who come in a popular or non-professional way' (Moriata, 1920: 4). Instigated by Franklin Roosevelt, the governor of New York State, who had himself taken a water cure for his polio, the new hydropathic establishment was opened in a state park adjoining the ancient springs in 1935 with massive bath houses dedicated to Franklin Roosevelt, Abraham Lincoln and George Washington and a research institute presided over by Dr Simon Baruch, Professor of Hydrotherapy at Columbia University and a leading advocate of the water cure. It was the most complete government health facility in the country with the capacity to treat over 4,500 patients a day. In its heyday between 1935 and 1960, it was attracting around 750,000 people a year.

The atmosphere in these new bathing establishments, as in Graefenberg and Wörishofen, where the hydropathic movement had begun, could not have been more different from that of the traditional spas. It was all health and no hedonism with the emphasis on wholesome outdoor pursuits and strenuous self-improvement rather than the self-indulgent indoor pleasures offered in stuffy, dimly lit casinos and ballrooms. Yet hydrotherapy was not without its influence on the European spa scene. The bracing cold douches, sitz baths and wet sheet packs advocated by Priessnitz and Kneipp were introduced as additional treatments in the bath houses of fashionable and long-established watering places. French *villes d'eaux* in particular enthusiastically adopted the cold douches which were known as 'Scotch showers'. In Aix-les-Bains around two thousand treatments involving high-pressure jets of cold water were being administered every summer by the 1840s (Plate 9). They were popularly dubbed 'the showers of hell' and described by one patient as resembling 'a liquid needle as thick as a man's arm' (Mackaman 1998: 111). Other treatments pioneered in hydros were also taken up, including vapour boxes and sealed steam baths to encourage sweating. If they gave a new boost to the serious medical aspect of traditional spas by introducing somewhat forbidding new treatments, they did not efface their hedonistic side, which was to have one last gloriously decadent flowering in La Belle Époque.

7

LA BELLE ÉPOQUE – THE FLOURISHING OF KARLSBAD AND MARIENBAD

During the closing decades of the nineteenth century and the opening years of the twentieth, Europe's spas blossomed and flourished in a glorious Indian summer with health and hedonism equally to the fore as an air of both decadence and desperation hung over the *Kurparks* and sanatoria. This period, known as La Belle Époque, sometimes dated as beginning with the end of the Franco-Prussian War in 1871, sometimes from 1890, and ending with the First World War, is associated with the final fling of the old European monarchies and aristocracy. This was certainly the case in the spas, perhaps most spectacularly in Karlsbad and Marienbad, which dominated this era, just as Bath did the eighteenth century and Baden-Baden the nineteenth. Other spas also went through a glorious renaissance, with a construction boom providing numerous new buildings in eclectic and extravagant architectural styles, ranging from neoclassical and Renaissance to oriental and art nouveau, complementing the fin-de-siècle atmosphere of the age. In several places casinos reopened as the bans on gambling were lifted and a number of prominent *Kurgäste*, led by the British king Edward VII, flirted outrageously and put *der Kurschatten* in its primary sense back at the heart of the spa experience.

It was not just the hedonistic aspects of spa life that flourished in La Belle Époque. With an increasingly middle-class clientele, which helped many spas achieve their highest ever number of guests in the 1890s and 1900s, there was also a renewed emphasis on the more serious healthy side, influenced partly by the hydrotherapy movement. Plenty of people still came to spas primarily to seek a cure and there were ever-growing numbers of doctors keen to take their money and treat them. One such was Dr Eduard Aronsohn who began practising in Bad Ems in 1889 and continued for twenty-five years. He published numerous case studies testifying to the efficacy of the waters there to cure disorders ranging from heart and circulatory conditions, through catarrh and bronchial complaints, to diseases of the kidneys and liver. They included one of a fifty-year-old Russian suffering from urinary calculus (stones in the bladder) who, 'afraid of an operation, came for a cure in Ems and four weeks later the stones were no longer there' and another of a satisfied male patient who said that 'he really had Ems to thank for his large family – in that his wife had used the uterus douche.' According to Dr Aronsohn, the Ems waters were equally effective in helping those seeking to gain weight and those wanting to lose it:

> A young, graceful baroness, circa 13 years old from Hungary came to Ems with suspected pulmonary apicitis and developed such a formidable appetite here that in five weeks she gained fourteen pounds; her loving mother on the other hand was anxious to lose weight, and indeed she lost fourteen pounds over the same period through a slimming cure. (Aronsohn 1912: 28)

This period saw a continuation of the medicalisation of spas, with increasing training for and specialisation by doctors. Laws were introduced in Germany and Austria-Hungary in the 1870s requiring all *Kurorte* to be under the control of university-trained physicians. Several individual spas became highly specialised in the diseases that they treated. By 1900, 70 per cent of the patients receiving treatments at Aix-la-Chapelle (Aachen), famous for its thermal sulphur baths, were syphilitics. More complex treatments were introduced, often based on new technology and using radiation and electricity, often in rather alarming-sounding procedures, such as the D'Arsonval High Frequency treatment, which involved passing electric currents through the patient while under water, and faradisation, galvanism and ionisation, which used electrodes soaked in weak solutions of various chemicals. There were also electric-light baths of various kinds in which patients sat or stood between heated panels or rows of light bulbs, sometimes with a spray douche being applied. From the 1890s onwards many spas developed private clinics offering these and other treatments, often tucked away on the edges of *Kurparks* and further segregating the sick from the more able *Kurgäste*. For the latter there were also exercise classes, the precursors of modern aerobics, Pilates and weight training. In 1897 the *Fremden-Blatt*, the weekly newspaper for guests at Bad Ragaz, among whom Germans and English predominated, advertised the newly established Institute for Swedish Gymnastics with its range of mechanical and aquatic aids to assist stretching, lifting and muscle toning. More traditional hedonistic attractions were not forgotten in this new emphasis on health. Perhaps in an attempt to appeal to the small but growing transatlantic clientele, the *Fremden-Blatt* also reminded guests that the daily *Kur* concerts offered Budweiser on draught and 'American drinks'.

Another new development was the growing tendency to take an 'after cure' in a sanatorium or convalescent boarding house which was often located away from the spa where the initial cure had been carried out. Isaac Burney Yeo, Professor of Medicine at King's College, London, who wrote a detailed compendium on *The Therapeutics of Mineral Springs and Climates* in 1904, noted this trend approvingly:

> It is certainly most undesirable, after a course of mineral waters and baths, to return at once to the cares and anxieties of business, or household management, or to fulfill social engagements. A period of calm and repose, in cheerful surroundings, is most useful in consolidating and confirming the good effects of bath treatment. (Yeo 1904: 50)

For British patients, this trend provided a welcome boost for seaside resorts, which were ideally placed to offer such facilities for post-spa recuperation. Yeo suggested that those coming back from treatment at a Continental spa 'select a resort conveniently placed on the homeward route, so as to divide the journey and lessen the fatigue of travelling'. He recommended several English south-coast resorts and also the original Spa in Belgium, conveniently sited on the route back from Germany 'with beautiful surroundings for drives and walks'.

This period also saw an increasing focus on psychological illnesses brought about by stress, the increasing pace and demands of life in more industrialised societies, and what would now be called burnout. The condition was widely referred to as 'neurasthenia'. Recognised symptoms included dizziness and fainting as well as general lassitude, depression and low spirits. Several spas came to specialise in treating this condition, notably Wiesbaden in Germany and a number of the southern French *villes d'eaux*. The French writer Octave Mirbeau based his novel *Les Vingt et un jours d'un neurasthénique* partly on his experience of taking a month-long cure in Luchon in the Pyrenees in 1897. It provides a grim picture of someone seeking relief from neurasthenia who journeys from sanatorium to asylum to desolate mountain retreat, subjecting himself to all sorts of new-fangled and frightening therapies and finding his fellow *curistes* universally unprepossessing: 'Amidst all these ugly visages and sagging bellies, I hardly ever experienced the surprise of seeing a pretty face or a thin frame!' Professor Yeo devoted considerable attention to neurasthenia, which he saw as encompassing hysteria, depression, neuralgia and nervous exhaustion. In addition to spa cures, he recommended those suffering from it to have 'recourse to picturesque mountain and lake regions in Switzerland, Italy or the Tyrol, or a yachting cruise in the Mediterranean, a winter tour in Egypt or Algiers, or visits to the historic cities of Southern Italy and Sicily' (Yeo 1904: 730). Here was an early medical endorsement of places that would prove significant and popular alternatives to spas in the later twentieth century. For the time being, however, Europe's *Kurorte* and *villes d'eaux* fought off the challenge of resorts sited amidst Alpine lakes and mountains or along the shores of the Mediterranean and held their own as the first choice for those seeking to alleviate stress and ill health through a combination of their water cures and their amusements and distractions.

The spas of Germany, France and Austria embarked on expensive and elaborate new building projects in the closing decades of the nineteenth century, boldly proclaiming their confidence in the future. In Baden-Baden there was no hint of the decline that had set in with the Franco-Prussian War when the magnificent Friedrichsbad (1877) was complemented by two more large bath houses, the Landesbad (1888) and the Kaiserin Augustabad, established for ladies only in 1890. In 1897 a state-of-the-art Inhalatorium was built to cater for patients with respiratory diseases undertaking the increasingly popular treatments involving inhalation of steam, gases and vapour baths. In Bad Homburg the Kaiser-Wilhelm-Bad was completed in 1890, with an Italian Renaissance exterior and Moorish mosaics adding to the Oriental atmosphere inside. Wiesbaden, where a new theatre opened in 1894, largely on the insistence of Kaiser Wilhelm II who went on to attend more than 100 performances there, was the last of the major German *Kurorte* to construct a new bath house in this period, with its Kaiser-Friedrich-Bad, erected in 1913. It also had one of the most impressive spa hotels, the Nassauer Hof, which opened in 1907 having taken ten years to build. Its 300 bedrooms were all equipped with private baths and a vast treatment complex, fed by its own thermal spring, which included Moorish baths, electric-light baths, alternating-current baths, steam baths, cold-water baths, suction and hot-air treatments, vibrating and pneumatic massages and electro-shock therapy. It also boasted a special chair for colonic irrigation which could pump a dozen litres of water through the colon in less than two minutes. Among the special features of the equally lavish Grand Hôtel de l'Europe in Bad

Gastein, Austria, opened in 1909, were urinals with specially placed mirrors so that stout gentlemen could admire their equipment.

The *villes d'eaux* in the Auvergne region of France, which also achieved their glory days in this period, were given particularly sumptuous and spectacular architectural makeovers. In Vichy, where the number of *curistes* mushroomed from 40,000 in 1900 to over 100,000 in 1914, the opulent Halle des Sources, a massive wrought-iron and glass pavilion built over the four main springs and resembling a giant greenhouse, dates from the 1890s. The Thermal Establishment was built in the same decade in Moorish style, its entrance crowned by an immense golden dome and the exterior walls decorated with glazed blue earthenware panels featuring mermaids and sirens. Inside mildly erotic pastel murals depict more mermaids, river nymphs and voluptuous female bathers. The dazzling polychromatic bath houses of Le Mont-Dore, designed to recreate the atmosphere of Roman *thermae* from the time of Diocletian, date from the same period. Adjoining its vast halls and galleries supported by marble pillars were the *salles de brouillard* where *curistes* sat on wooden benches in an atmosphere of thick mist or inhaled thermal gases from lengths of rubber tubing. The architecture of nearby La Bourboule, where the main thermal establishment was built in Moorish style in 1872 along the banks of the Dordogne, reflected the more hedonistic aspects of spa life. No less than four casinos were built here during La Belle Époque, including a special Casino des Enfants to cater for the large number of children who took treatments there for asthma.

The spas of the Auvergne were much frequented by writers and feature in several novels of this period. Mimi, the heroine of Lidia Veselitskaia's *Mimochka*, takes a cure in Vichy in the 1890s. Le Mont-Dore's regular visitors included Marcel Proust, Anatole France (who made it the setting for his 1879 novel *Jocaste*) and George Sand, who took twelve cures there towards the end of her life and has the character of Raphaël Personnaz in her *Jean de la Roche* take the waters in an effort to promote longevity. Émile Zola spent the month of August 1884 in Le Mont-Dore with his wife, taking baths and long walks. It was the only break he had during the period of composition of his novel *Germinal*. It was during his regular visits to take the waters in Châtel-Guyon in the 1880s that Guy de Maupassant gained inspiration for his novel *Mont-Oriol* about the creation of a new spa in the Auvergne region.

This was also a boom time for ostentatious building projects in British spas, even though they were in clear decline and the biggest and grandest hotels were now to be found in seaside resorts. The Royal Baths at Harrogate were opened in 1897 providing sumptuously opulent Turkish baths with beautiful Moorish designs. The same year saw the building of the adjoining Winter Gardens which are now, alas, a vast and vulgar Wetherspoons pub. In Buxton a new pump room opened in 1894 and the hot baths were extended several times during the 1890s. Facilities for recreation and culture were also greatly improved with the magnificent new Opera House, designed by Frank Matcham, opened in 1903. In the same year a *Kursaal*, also designed by Matcham and incorporating a theatre, was opened in Harrogate. It was renamed 'The Royal Hall' on the outbreak of the First World War and so it has remained, although its original German name is still evident on top of the façade, making it the only *Kursaal* in Britain. Amid this prevailing and rather decadent opulence, it is perhaps refreshing to note that in the tiny Welsh spa of Llandrindod Wells the main public building erected in this period was the Albert Hall, built in 1896 to seat nearly 700 people and primarily used for the visitors' prayer meetings every weekday morning. As a historian of the town rightly notes, this was 'a feature of Llandrindod life that made it unique among spas' (Jones 1975: 15).

Although it was hardly on the scale of what the Nonconformist conscience contributed to the urban landscape of Llandrindod Wells, British guests did bring some wholesome influences to bear on the physical layout and ambience of several Continental spas. As well as planting Anglican churches in many of the most fashionable watering places, they were largely responsible for introducing healthy outdoor games like tennis, golf and football which flourished for a time following the prohibition of gambling in German *Kurorte* in the early 1870s. All three games were introduced in Baden-Baden by Archibald White, vicar of the Anglican Church of All Saints which had been established there in 1867 to cater for the growing number of English-speaking guests. The tennis club which he founded in 1881, the first in Germany, is still to be found in the Lichtentaler Allee, its courts pointedly sited just opposite the French gardens. Marienbad also gained tennis courts the same year, the first in the Austro-Hungarian Empire. The equipment for the game came from England, with the racquets being allowed through Austrian customs on the basis that they were some new kind of musical instrument. With the resumption of gambling in many Continental spas, the appeal of these more manly and healthy outdoor sports somewhat declined, although horse racing flourished, providing inveterate gamblers with a form of betting which did not involve long nights in stuffy casinos.

Although they may have played a small but significant role in bringing moral uplift and muscular Christianity to Continental spas with their healthy outdoor games, British guests were not immune from or averse to the more traditional spa sport of flirting and the lure of the *Kurschatten*. Englishmen visiting Bad Ems were renowned for loading pretty young ladies into wheelbarrows and racing them through the woods. They were not alone in engaging in this kind of activity. The growing popularity of cycling provided new opportunities for amorous dalliances in the shady wooded areas around spa towns. One who took full advantage of them was the Austrian author and dramatist, Arthur Schnitzler, who enjoyed invigorating trysts with lady cyclists in the woods around Ischl. Other *Kurgäste* took a more restrained and chivalrous approach to their flirting, like Prince Proworoff, secretary of state to the Russian tsar, who became known in Bad Ems as '*Der Rosenkavalier*' because of his habit during his frequent stays there of walking down the promenade every morning with two dozen roses which he distributed among the most beautiful ladies that he encountered. There were also those who appear to have obtained their sexual thrills from the treatments they took. This seems to have been true for the French poet Paul Verlaine, not usually one to shun casual sexual encounters, when he took a cure to try to mitigate the effects of gonorrhea, syphilis, diabetes and cirrhosis of the liver in Aix-les-Bains in 1889. Arrested on his arrival for being drunk, he was too raddled with his addiction to absinthe and drugs to be capable of any sexual activity. He noted that while 'the water is hot, slightly sulphurous and unpleasant', his massages were 'almost voluptuous' and they apparently gave him enough pleasure to inspire the highly erotic poems which he wrote during his cure.

Aix seems to have had quite a reputation for amorous activity in the 1890s. An 1896 novel set there, *Le Médecin des Dames de Néans* by René Boylesve, centres around the seduction of an older woman by a young man. Madame Durosay, the bored wife of a provincial notary, is sent by her doctor, who feels that she needs a new lover, to take the waters at Aix accompanied by her husband and a vigorous young blood, Septime de Jallais. She enjoys a suitably steamy relationship with Septime there while her husband also manages to engage in a satisfying tryst with a fellow *curiste*. Another novel set in Aix, *L'Âme Étrangère* (1894) by Guy de Maupassant, describes similar amorous goings-on and provides a less than flattering pen portrait of the spa:

> This city of showers and casinos, of hygiene and pleasure, in which all the princes of the earth whom thrones have rejected fraternized with all the *Rastaquouères* [foreign upstarts and interlopers] whom prisons did not wish to hold ... this unique salad of worldly and funny people, dining at the neighbouring tables, speaking aloud of each other, and playing, an hour later, elbow-to-elbow around the same carpet. (Maupassant 1910: 152)

The leading German *Kurorte* similarly maintained their reputation for cosmopolitan decadence, as testified in this description of

Baden-Baden around 1900 by the British diplomat, Horace Rumbold:

> In the motley crowd that thronged the broad walk, or sat in closely packed rows round the kiosk where the band was playing, or lounged by the shop of Millerio the jeweller, or flirted and tattled at the tables under the trees, every type and class and nation was represented. We had here a perfect epitome of European society in all its shades and gradations: German royalty, French art and literature, Parisian fashion and frailty; the greatest ladies from London, Vienna, and St Petersburg cheek by jowl with the fairest sinners from Berlin or the Quartier Breda; the impassive *croupier* and the fevered, broken gambler side by side; English black-legs jostling Frankfurt Jew stockbrokers; lanky Baden dragoons mixed with the stalwart Croats of *Benedek infanterie* and the boyish looking recruits of the Prussian regiments ...
>
> It was a gaudy, bewildering, yet strangely intoxicating scene – essentially of the earth earthy – but set in such lovely surroundings, that when the soft moon stole over it from above the ruins of the *Alte Schloss*, tipping the tall trees with silver and marking their shadows on the quiet lawns and walks beyond, one could only revel in its singular beauty, and he must have been a churl indeed, or a pedant, who could moralize over, instead of giving himself wholly up to, its magic charm. (Rumbold 1902: 227–8)

No European spa in La Belle Époque, not even Baden-Baden, had quite the cachet or reputation of the Bohemian duo of Karlsbad and Marienbad. Their rise had a lot to do with the fact that they were not in Germany where the *Kurorte* became increasingly regimented, prim and Prussian under the rule of Kaiser Wilhelm II, who succeeded to the imperial throne in 1888. Karlsbad was the first to challenge the long dominance of the German spas. Among its earliest visitors in this era was Karl Marx who made three visits in the mid-1870s. A lifelong hypochondriac, he was plagued by liver complaints, spells of dizziness, frequent headaches and insomnia. After a three-week cure in Harrogate, he was urged by his London doctor to try Karlsbad and he went there in 1874 with his nineteen-year-old daughter Eleanor, nicknamed Tussy, a chronic invalid who was refusing to eat and spitting up blood. He travelled there under the pseudonym of 'Charles Marx, squire of London' in an attempt to avert police suspicions at a time when his name was being linked with riots across Europe. In fact, the police were well aware of his presence but after keeping him under surveillance for a month they concluded that he gave no cause for suspicion. Both he and Tussy concentrated on the cure, as he reported to his friend Friedrich Engels:

> We are both living in strict accordance with the rules. We go to our respective springs at six every morning, where I have to drink seven glasses. Between each two glasses there has to be a break of 15 minutes during which one marches up and down. After the last glass, an hour's walk, and finally coffee. Another cold glass in the evening before bed. (Wheen 1999: 357)

Somewhat surprisingly, Marx seems to have proved himself the life and soul of the *Kurgäste* during his stays at Karlsbad. A Viennese newspaper reported that 'he always had to hand the *mot juste*, the striking simile, the suddenly illuminating joke' (Wheen 1999: 358). Although he found his three cures there helpful in easing his various conditions, he subsequently switched to the small Rhineland spa of Bad Neuenahr. He was put off by the pollution in Karlsbad with its extensive logging and mining industries and coal burning, which he complained turned the air into 'a brownish yellow colour'. Augustus Granville had earlier commented on another unsatisfactory feature of its environment, the prominent position at the end of the promenade of the ladies' and gentlemen's toilets 'which, by their incessant opening and shutting, proclaim the active influence of the saline beverage'. He pleaded that they might be placed 'out of sight, as well as out of the reach of the olfactory organs' (Granville 2012: 104).

A detailed account of Karlsbad in its heyday is provided by the American author William Dean Howells, whose 1886 novel *Their Silver Wedding Journey* describes a Mr and Mrs March taking a cure there. March is portrayed as a classic hypochondriac. He is convinced that his symptoms of depression and gloom come from his liver and as his wife says, 'Carlsbad is the great place for that.' When he gets there he is rather disappointed to learn that he is not as ill as he thought he was:

> March sat with a company of other patients in the anteroom of the doctor, and when it came his turn to be prodded and kneaded, he was ashamed at being told he was not so bad a case as he had dreaded. The doctor wrote out a careful dietary for him, with a prescription of a certain number of glasses of water at a certain spring and a certain number of baths, and a rule for the walks he was to take before and after eating; then the doctor patted him on the shoulder and pushed him caressingly out of his inner office. It was too late to begin his treatment that day, but he went with his wife to buy a cup, with a strap for hanging it over his shoulder, and he put it on so as to be an invalid with the others at once.

The description of the atmosphere at the springs as March begins his cure is worth quoting at some length:

> At five the next morning he rose, and on his way to the street exchanged with the servants cleaning the hotel stairs the first of the gloomy '*Guten Morgens*' which usher in the day at Carlsbad. They cannot be so finally hopeless as they sound; they are probably expressive only of the popular despair of getting through with them before night; but March heard the salutations sorrowfully groaned out on every hand as he joined the straggling current

of invalids which swelled on the way past the silent shops and cafés in the Alte Wiese, till it filled the street, and poured its thousands upon the promenade before the classic colonnade of the Muhlbrunn. On the other bank of the Tepl the Sprudel flings its steaming waters by irregular impulses into the air under a pavilion of iron and glass; but the Muhlbrunn is the source of most resort. There is an instrumental concert somewhere in Carlsbad from early rising till bedtime; and now at the Muhlbrunn there was an orchestra already playing; and under the pillared porch, as well as before it, the multitude shuffled up and down, draining their cups by slow sips, and then taking each his place in the interminable line moving on to replenish them at the spring.

A picturesque majority of Polish Jews, whom some vice of their climate is said peculiarly to fit for the healing effects of Carlsbad, most took his eye in their long gabardines of rusty black and their derby hats of plush or velvet, with their corkscrew curls coming down before their ears. They were old and young, they were grizzled and red and black, but they seemed all well-to-do; and what impresses one first and last at Carlsbad is that its waters are mainly for the healing of the rich. After the Polish Jews, the Greek priests of Russian race were the most striking figures. There were types of Latin ecclesiastics, who were striking in their way too; and the uniforms of certain Austrian officers and soldiers brightened the picture. Here and there a southern face, Italian or Spanish or Levantine, looked passionately out of the mass of dull German visages; for at Carlsbad the Germans, more than any other gentile nation, are to the fore. Their misfits, their absence of style, imparted the prevalent effect; though now and then among the women a Hungarian, or Pole, or Parisian, or American, relieved the eye which seeks beauty and grace rather than the domestic virtues.

At the springs, a line of young girls with a steady mechanical action dipped the cups into the steaming source, and passed them impersonally up to their owners. With the patients at the

Muhlbrunn it was often a half-hour before one's turn came, and at all a strict etiquette forbade any attempt to anticipate it. The water was merely warm and flat, and after the first repulsion one could forget it. March formed a childish habit of counting ten between the sips, and of finishing the cup with a gulp which ended it quickly; he varied his walks between cups by going sometimes to a bridge at the end of the colonnade where a group of Triestines were talking Venetian, and sometimes to the little Park beyond the Kurhaus, where some old women were sweeping up from the close sward the yellow leaves which the trees had untidily dropped overnight. He liked to sit there and look at the city beyond the Tepl, where it climbed the wooded heights in terraces till it lost its houses in the skirts and folds of the forest. (Howells 2006, Part 2, Chapter 28)

As portrayed by Howells, Karlsbad is just as cosmopolitan as Baden-Baden but more focused on the cure and more sedate and genteel. It also has that distinctive air of unreality that hangs over all spas. March felt it as he walked through the woods: 'The other invalids who haunted the forest, and passed up and down before him in fulfilment of their several prescriptions, had a thin unreality in spite of the physical bulk that prevailed among them.' But more than anything else it is the demureness and douceness of the place that comes across in the pages of *Their Silver Wedding Journey*. No mention here of late-night gambling or carousing:

By nine o'clock everything is hushed; not a wheel is heard at that dead hour; the few feet shuffling stealthily through the Alte Wiese whisper a caution of silence to those issuing with a less guarded tread from the opera; the little bowers that overhang the stream are as dark and mute as the restaurants across the way which serve meals in them by day; the whole place is as forsaken as other cities at midnight. People get quickly home to bed, or if they have a mind to snatch a belated joy, they slip into the Theater-Café, where the sleepy Frauleins serve them, in an exemplary drowse, with plates of cold ham and bottles of the gently gaseous waters of Giesshubl. (Howells 2006, Part 2, Chapter 34)

Karlsbad's popularity and opulence during La Belle Époque is very evident from the exuberant proliferation of ornate buildings which date from this period and which still today give the whole place the appearance of a set for some Ruritanian opera. The French architect Le Corbusier described the effect as being like 'a gathering of cakes' – very creamy and fancy ones, one might add. Many of these buildings, which range in style between neoclassical, neo-baroque, neo-Renaissance and art nouveau, have been recently restored. They include three of the drinking colonnades housing the twelve main springs: the stone Mlýnská (Mill) Colonnade (1871–2); the wrought-iron Sadový (Park) Colonnade (1881); and the wooden Tržní (Market) Colonnade (1883, extended 1904); and also the theatre (1884–6); the Grandhotel Pupp (1893); the Imperial Bath House built on the site of a brewery in 1895; the Alžbětiny Lázně (Elizabeth Baths), a vast balneological facility named after Franz Joseph's wife and built in 1906; and the massive Hotel Imperial (1910–12) which towers over the town like some Disneyland fairy castle.

Marienbad, which was to establish a rather racier if equally fashionable and elegant reputation, underwent a similar building boom in the last two decades of the nineteenth century. The magnificent cast-iron colonnade, which still dominates the central spa area of the town, was erected in 1889. The old and new spa buildings (now the Centrální Lázně and Nové Lázně hotels), equipped with the latest in gas baths and bathing equipment and inspired by the architecture of the French Riviera, followed in the early 1890s and a *Kurhaus* was erected between them in 1900. Around the central *Kurpark* vast hotels in over-the-top neo-baroque- and neo-Renaissance-style sprouting towers, turrets and putti were erected to cater for the numerous rich and famous patrons coming to escape the increasing constrictions and severities of the German *Kurorte*. Not all of them liked what they found there. Friedrich Nietzsche spent two months in Marienbad in 1880 in an attempt to curb his chronic migraines. He found that taking the water made his headaches worse, the people were 'so ugly' and the food very expensive, and complained that 'it is like being in an evil world.' Even the fact that his great hero Goethe had loved Marienbad failed to convince him of its charms. He noted on leaving that Goethe seemed never to have had a single profound thought while there, and it had been the same for him. Sigmund Freud found Marienbad equally unsatisfactory when he sought a cure for gastrointestinal troubles. The atmosphere simply provoked melancholia. He preferred Karlsbad which he visited five times between 1910 and 1915. Stefan Zweig, whose annual visits to Marienbad with his parents so that his mother could seek relief from her many maladies provided the basis for his story of spa seduction, 'The Burning Secret' (see page 16), found the atmosphere similarly oppressive and febrile. Mark Twain, too, was discomforted by a stay there in 1890. He had gone primarily just to observe the scene but it was not long before he had succumbed to the prevailing ambience of hypochondria and morbid introspection 'and pretty soon I was a good deal concerned about myself'. He dutifully started drinking 'the dreadful water', eating 'only the food I didn't want' and having a generally miserable time, reflecting 'I don't see any advantage in this over having the gout.' He found the spa regime over-regulated and oppressive: 'they make you drop everything that gives an interest to life.' When at the end of his stay he was told that he was free from disease, he tartly commented: 'What I have been through in these two weeks would free a person of pretty much everything in him that wasn't nailed down there.'

In contrast to these negative reactions, several of the many British visitors to Marienbad seem to have had a thoroughly good experience. The Liberal politician Henry Campbell-Bannerman went there annually from 1876 to 1906, staying for six weeks or more, chiefly for the benefit of his wife, who had indifferent health. Another regular visitor was John, later Lord Fisher, who as Admiral of the Fleet and First Sea Lord, is generally regarded as the most important figure in British naval history after Nelson. His memoirs provide a delightful account of how he first came to go there in 1889 in an effort to relieve the effects of dysentery which had plagued him for many years:

> When all the doctors failed to cure me, I accidentally came across a lovely partner I used to waltz with, who begged me to go to Marienbad in Bohemia. I did so, and in three weeks I was in robust health. It was the Pool of Bethesda, and this waltzing angel put me into it, for it really was a miracle, and I never again had a recurrence of my illness. (Fisher 1919: 157)

It was Edward VII who really put Marienbad on the map both as the spa to go to, and to be seen at, and as the perfect place for engaging in amorous dalliances. He first went there as Prince of Wales in 1897, returning two years later. His impact on its popularity and its reputation was instantaneous, as Campbell-Bannerman noted with some distaste:

> We have seen a new realization of the saying that 'wheresoever the eagle is there will the carcasses be gathered together'. Whether on account of the Prince's presence or not, the English and American society here has contained an extraordinary number of tainted ladies – including five divorcées and about ten others of various degrees of doubtfulness. The decent people were almost in a minority and we thought of wearing our marriage certificates as a sort of order on our coats. (Wilson 1973: 143)

For much of his time as Prince of Wales, Edward had favoured Bad Homburg, finding that its waters and regime helped in his lifelong struggle to reduce weight. During one two-week stay there he managed to shed forty pounds, partly through vigorous games of tennis, despite starting the day with a champagne breakfast and ending it with a champagne supper at the casino. Despite his efforts, his girth remained substantial, earning him the nickname Tum-Tum, and he was unable to do up the bottom button of his waistcoat, creating a fashion which persists to this day. He started another fashion by favouring what became known as the Homburg hat. He was an enthusiastic patron of the Bad Homburg casino before it closed as part of the general German clampdown on gambling. He also enjoyed several trysts there, starting on his very first visit in 1882 when, aged forty-one, he pursued the nineteen-year-old daughter of an American railroad tycoon. During his stay in 1893 Edward helped to rescue a fellow British *Kurgast*, the Earl of Rosebery, from being pursued by the Marquess of Queensberry, father of Oscar Wilde's lover, Lord Alfred Douglas. Convinced that Rosebery was having an affair with his eldest son, Lord Drumlanrig, Queensberry came to Homburg determined to expose 'that boy pimp and boy lover'. Edward intervened and sent the homophobic Marquess back home, telling him 'we are quiet people at Homburg and don't like disturbance.'

In fact, Homburg became rather too quiet and staid for Edward's taste. He found its heavy Prussian atmosphere increasingly oppressive and resented the way that his nephew Kaiser Wilhelm II kept subjecting him to military parades and disapproving lectures about the state of his morals. As king, he made Marienbad his main summer retreat, going there under the name of the Duke of Lancaster, and staying for three or four weeks every year from 1903 to 1907. His reputation as Edward the Caresser attracted a number of ladies of easy virtue who journeyed there in the hope of catching his eye. They included the actress Lily Langtry, who had been his mistress in the 1880s and 90s. Now greying and considerably past her prime, she was, in his biographer Gordon Brook-Shepherd's words, 'a reminder of romance rather than an invitation to it'. Another suitor, discreetly referred to as Mrs X, who was in her thirties, was a more exciting prospect and, as well as visiting her in her house, the king regularly took her for a ride in a carriage and pair to a café situated in a dairy tucked away in the woods outside the town. Although he was able to dismiss his equerry, he was not able to shake off the Austrian police commissioner detailed to protect him. This attentive guard followed in another carriage at a discreet distance and wandered around in the woods while the king and his lady friend were in the dairy. Eventually Mrs X was supplanted in the king's affection by an American actress. Mrs X promptly left by car for Germany with a 'certain Foreign Minister' at whose side she was seen throughout the rest of the season at Baden-Baden.

Edward VII's popularity with ladies was such that, in the words of Brook-Shepherd, 'candidates for his favours took to turning up in Marienbad, as though they were applying for an official post'. One Viennese beauty appeared at the office of his private secretary, Frederick Ponsonby, at the end of a long line of official interviewees and announced that she wanted to have the honour of sleeping with the king. Ponsonby replied that this was out of the question, whereupon she suggested that in order not to waste her train fare she might as well go to bed with the king's secretary instead. A somewhat embarrassed Ponsonby declined her offer, whereupon she got up and left in a huff. Ponsonby had to deal with several ladies of similar dubious repute who gathered around the king. He described one faded Parisian beauty as possessing 'an eye glass, short skirts and a murky past' (Brook-Shepherd 1975: 213). Like Goethe and Chopin, Edward VII seems to have succumbed to the aphrodisiac effects of Marienbad's famous love spring, although he hardly needed such stimulation, and could be seen pursuing young ladies around the *Kurpark*. He was particularly taken by one who made and sold hats under the colonnade. In the diplomatically chosen words of Sigmund Münz, an Austrian journalist who covered the king's visits to Marienbad and subsequently wrote a book about them, 'from time to time he was kind enough to buy one of her hats, which she had to deliver to him personally at the hotel' (Münz 1934: 24).

EdwardVII took rooms in theWeimar Hotel, described as 'a cross in style between a baroque Bohemian shooting-lodge and a French provincial opera house'. His five-room suite included a study where a large oil painting hung over his writing-desk depicting a scene entitled *Solitude*. It could hardly have been less appropriate given his lifestyle there. He entertained lavishly in the hotel, with dinners often featuring grouse from Balmoral, his favourite vegetable of *aubergines frites*, and peaches for dessert, and held somewhat risqué parties, at one of which Maud Allan, an English dancer, appeared clad only in 'two oyster shells and a five-franc piece'. Although he was hardly a model of propriety in his own dealings with women, he adopted a distinctly puritanical tone when it came to public performances. When a recital by a well-known Austrian cabaret singer included a skit in which a licentious Catholic priest took off his robes at the request of a voluptuous countess, Edward walked out in disgust and the singer was dispatched back to Vienna with a heavy fine. He walked out on another occasion in 1907 when a touring cabaret appearing in the local theatre sang a series of lewd songs. When news of this reached England, the bishop of London sent the king a fulsome letter praising his Christian stand against obscenity. He told his secretary to reply to the bishop that 'I have no wish to pose as protector of morals, especially abroad.'

Edward VII's antics in Marienbad both intrigued and worried diplomats and politicians. The Austro-Hungarian ambassador to Russia reported that when the English king met Count Izvolsky, the Russian foreign minister, and Georges Clemenceau, the French prime minister, both regular *Kurgäste* at Marienbad, their conversation was almost entirely about Edward's amatory adventures. 'Politics have been completely relegated to the background,' the ambassador went on to complain, 'and erotics have reigned exclusively' (Münz 1934: 52). Campbell-Bannerman continued to be in a state of moral frenzy about the effects of his monarch's reputation and the kind of people he attracted. 'We have the great man here with a cloud of bluebottle flies buzzing around him,' he wrote from Marienbad in 1904. 'It is worse than ever – he is recklessly abandoned to the society of a few semi-déclassé ladies and men to match' (Wilson 1973: 143). During an earlier stay he had complained to W. E. Gladstone's son Herbert: 'In this small society of English people, quite half of the ladies either have already been, or are qualifying themselves for being, divorced: and a considerable number of the men are helping.' Their antics, he said, had given the English 'an evil name for scandals and loose living such as the poor Austrians (who do not pretend to much morality) have never seen equalled. Lords and ladies and others have no right to come out to a quiet place like this and disgrace their country' (Wilson 1973: 142).

Alongside his evident enjoyment of the more hedonistic side of spa life, Edward VII does seem to have been quite assiduous in taking the waters during the seven summers that he spent in Marienbad. He went to drink at one of the main springs early every morning, sometimes at the Elisabeth Brunnen, named after his great-aunt Elizabeth, princess of Hesse-Homburg and daughter of George III, and regularly bathed in the Nové Lázně, or New Baths. The royal spa cabin constructed for him there remains largely unaltered today and can still be booked by guests staying at the Nové Lázně hotel. Richly decorated with tiles and pillars in Oriental style, and designed to evoke the atmosphere of the tales of the *Arabian Nights*, it contained a special armchair with a carefully concealed set of scales which allowed the king to be weighed as he sat in it. He described his daily regime in a letter during his 1905 stay: 'I appear at the Kreuzbrunnen at 7.30 and get through three tumblers of the rather pleasant water by 9, when *le café au lait* is very welcome. Luncheon at one, dinner at 7.30. Bridge frequently but always to bed by 11' (Brook-Shepherd 1975: 218). Although it sounds abstemious, this regime involved gargantuan meals and much entertaining and it nearly finished off Campbell-Bannerman who spent much time with the king during that particular stay. On Edward's departure, he took to his bed for forty-eight hours exhausted by the royal energy and appetite. As

Münz observed, while most *Kurgäste* were under medical orders to give up women, wine and song, 'the only thing the King seemed to drop temporarily was wine. This he replaced by the alkaline waters of the *Kreuzbrunnen*. But women and song were things he did not want to miss at Marienbad' (Münz 1934: 58). Edward maintained his philandering right up to his last visit in 1907 when at the age of sixty-six he took up with a forty-one-year-old American actress, Maxine Elliott, whom he had met in Marienbad the previous year when she had come out specially to catch his eye, strategically positioning herself on a bench which she knew he always passed on his morning walk. He entertained her at least four times to lunch – she shared his passion for food and was known to eat large quantities of butter without bread – and as his biographer, Jane Ridley, comments, 'who knows what went on in the afternoons behind closed curtains in her scented hotel room?' (Ridley 2012: 438).

For all the rather racy and louche reputation that Edward VII's visits helped to give it, Marienbad also presented a more demure and serious aspect. Indeed, as described by Sigmund Münz, there was an almost sacred atmosphere around the springs early every morning during the season:

> Anyone rising early in the middle of summer and making his way to the *Brunnen* – say between 5 and 6 am – might think he was witnessing the celebration of some holy rite. The morning half-light showed black figures slowly drifting along like pilgrims, reaching out eagerly for their cups, and then slowly sipping – all giving an impression of rapt devotion. (Münz 1934: 22)

This impression was enhanced by the presence of monks from the nearby abbey of Teplá, which continued to own the springs, who appeared in white cassocks and black top hats, together with Polish and Russian Jews, with their long beards and side curls, dressed in long kaftans and looking 'as if they had met for morning prayer', their faces bearing 'an expression of melancholy'.

Karlsbad and Marienbad both achieved the height of their popularity in the years immediately before the outbreak of the First World War. The number of *Kurgäste* at Karlsbad peaked at 70,935 in 1911 and Marienbad welcomed its highest ever number of guests (34,509) in the same year. Other spas also flourished in this period, constructing buildings of ever greater extravagance and eccentricity, like the Buddhist Temple in the middle of the *Kurpark* in Bad Homburg given by King Chulalongkorn of Siam in 1907 in gratitude for a successful cure, and the casino built in Évian in 1912 on the model of the Basilica of St Sophia in Istanbul. Grand bath houses and hotels continued to be erected right up to the outbreak of the war and even during it. In Budapest the vast Széchenyi Baths, the first thermal baths to be built on the Pest side of the Danube and the largest of their kind in Europe, were constructed between 1909 and 1913 in what the guidebooks refer to as a 'modern Renaissance' style, but I would be inclined to categorise rather as neo-Biedermeier baroque with orange-coloured walls and lots of domes, pillars and galleries. Over the same period detailed plans were made for a magnificent spa hotel adjoining and incorporating the historic Gellért thermal baths on the other (Buda) bank of the river. The Gellért Hotel was not in fact completed until 1918. A massive art deco structure, capped by huge domes and turrets with much use inside of coloured glass, sweeping staircases, arcades and balconies, the whole complex was bombed by the Allies in January 1945 but hastily rebuilt and still stands today as a confident expression of the exuberance and vitality of the spa scene in the last days of the Austro-Hungarian Empire.

There are even hints of Europe's royalty and aristocracy enjoying a final fling in the rather more faded and restrained elegance of the English spas in their Edwardian sunset years. A plaque on the wall of Cathcart House on the parade in Harrogate records a tea party there in 1911 attended by Empress Marie of Russia, Queen Alexandra, widow of Edward VII, King Manuel of Spain, Prince Christopher of Greece and Grand Duchess Maria Georgievna of Russia. The

Grand Duchess, who regularly visited the Yorkshire spa with her sick daughter, Princess Xenia, was stranded there on the outbreak of the First World War in 1914. Told that it was too dangerous to return to Russia, she made herself useful by setting up a hospital for wounded servicemen which she ran with Princess Victoria, daughter of Queen Victoria, and Princess Margaret of Denmark. She later commandeered spa buildings to set up two more hospitals.

The lonely and melancholy introspection which was so much a part of the darker, hidden, shadow side of spa life did not disappear during the years of La Belle Époque. It is well brought out in Katherine Mansfield's set of short stories *In a German Pension*, published in 1911 and based on her own experience in Wörishofen where she had been packed off by her mother in 1909. In one of the stories a German *Kurgast* expresses incredulity at the reluctance of the English to engage in the favourite topic of conversation in all spas: 'You do not seem to enjoy discussing the functions of the body. As well speak of a railway train and refuse to mention the engine. How can we hope to understand anybody, knowing nothing of their stomachs?' Another story features the bizarre characters who inhabit the Luft Bad, a 'collection of plain wooden cells' where patients come to breathe the air. One, whom Mansfield dubs 'the Vegetable Lady', informs her that she is making her own cure and living entirely on raw vegetables and nuts. The strange practices of another, who virtually lives in the Luft Bad, are described by a fellow guest: 'he buries himself up to the armpits in mud and refuses to believe in the Trinity.' There is also the inevitable story involving a *Kurschatten* when one of the *Kurgäste*, Violet, fantasises about a handsome man who comes into her room looking for someone else as she is contemplating ending her life by sinking her head into a full washbasin. As his figure rises before her, she cries out: 'There's a fount of happiness in me, that is drying up, little by little, in this hateful existence. I'll be dead if this goes on … I want passion, and love, and adventure – I yearn for them. Why should I stay here and rot?' (Mansfield 1995: 17, 43, 72).

The diaries of an earlier eminent Victorian visitor to Europe's spas give an even more poignant picture of their crushing dullness and capacity to instil an enervating sense of desperation. The composer Arthur Sullivan suffered for much of his life from excruciating pain in his kidneys, probably caused by stones, and it was in an attempt to gain some relief from this that he took his first spa cure in the summer of 1891 at Contrexéville. He was prescribed baths at 7 a.m. and 3 p.m. and four glasses of water between 8 and 9 a.m. For the rest of the day he took walks, played a little tennis, took occasional carriage rides, visited the theatre in the evenings and indulged his passion for gambling, proudly recording his winnings in the card game baccarat. Despite these distractions, his overwhelming sensation was one of boredom (see page 21) and he was uncertain as to the efficacy of the cure, noting that after thirty days of it, 'I still have the same pains as before'. Five years later, while staying in the Swiss lakeside resort of Lucerne, he succumbed to a classic *Kurschatten* in the form of a brief but total infatuation with a much younger woman. It led the fifty-four-year-old composer to propose to the twenty-two-year-old Violet Beddington. He told her that he thought he only had two years to live and would leave her everything when he died. She turned him down and subsequently married the novelist Sydney Schiff (pseudonym Stephen Hudson) who based a chapter of his 1925 novel, *Myrtle*, on the romance between Sullivan and Violet. His novel is set in Aix-les-Bains where an ailing composer has come after 'a round of German *bads*' in an attempt to cure diabetes.

It was, in fact, to Bad Gastein that Sullivan next resorted in 1898 in an attempt to alleviate his chronic kidney complaint. Despite the pleasure of having Lord Rosebery and other British aristocrats as fellow cure guests, he was bored by the regime, which included daily baths and massages and the application of a hot potato poultice on both thighs from 10 p.m. to 3 a.m. At the end of his stay he confided to his diary: 'My stay of three weeks at Gastein has been very quiet and I think very beneficial. I feel much fresher and better. The place itself is beautifully situated but dull and expensive.' His last spa cure was undertaken nearer home, at Tunbridge Wells, in October 1900, by which time his health had considerably worsened. On his first night, after having dinner, he felt his old pain coming on and 'in half an hour I was writhing and bathed in sweat.' He summoned a doctor who gave him an injection which provided instant relief and ensured a good night's rest. Although he felt a little better by the end of his stay, this solitary spa retreat left him with the classic *Kurgast*'s introspection: 'I have been here just a fortnight and what have I done? Little more than nothing, first from illness and physical incapacity, secondly from brooding and nervous terror about myself' (Bradley 2010: 20). That was the last but one entry in his diary. His condition deteriorated rapidly, he returned to London and died a month later.

The kind of music in which Sullivan excelled and with which he will for ever be associated, the light, lilting, lyrical melodies of comic opera and operetta, provided a soundtrack for Europe's spas throughout La Belle Époque. Selections from Savoy operas were played in *Kurkonzerte* along with compositions by Jacques Offenbach and Johann Strauss, the two other leading figures in what is often called the golden age of operetta who were frequent visitors to spas and did so much for their vibrant musical life. During this golden age, Baden bei Wien took on the role of the unofficial operetta capital of Europe. As we have already observed, it was almost certainly the setting for *Die Fledermaus* (see page 31). Among the operetta composers who made it their home were Karl Millöcker, who wrote *Der Bettelstudent* there in 1882, Carl Zeller, composer of *Der Vogelhändler*, and Karel Komzák, who conducted the *Kurorchester* and wrote a string of marches and waltzes celebrating the town with titles like *Badener Madl'n* and *Mein Baden*. All three met untimely ends in the town. Zeller died of pneumonia at the age of fifty-six in 1898, having never recovered from the physical and mental illness that assailed him after slipping on ice three years earlier. Millöcker died at the age of fifty-seven in 1899 and Komzak was only fifty-four when he fell under the wheels of a departing train at Baden station on Easter Sunday 1905. By then, the town, which was attracting over 30,000 *Kurgäste* a year, was establishing itself as a leading centre for operetta performance as well as composition. In 1906 the 657-seater Sommerarena with retractable roof was built over the original Roman springs to house open-air summer productions and the imposing Stadttheater was built the following year. Both remain leading venues for operetta performances. Arthur Schnitzler's 1911 play, *Das Weite Land*, which chronicles the multiple infidelities of a Viennese light-bulb manufacturer and his wife, was set in Baden bei Wien and confirmed its reputation as 'the grand theatre of the world', a real-life operetta stage on which romantic affairs were played out.

The silver age of operetta, which succeeded the golden age and began in the late 1900s, centred on another Austrian *Kurort*, Bad Ischl. Its leading figures, Franz Lehár, Oscar Straus, Leo Fall, Robert Stolz and Emmerich Kálmán, who composed music of a darker, more passionate and bitter-sweet character than the lighter, bouncier, more satirical works of Sullivan, Offenbach and Strauss, were all regular summer visitors there. So were their less well-known contemporaries like Rudi Gfaller, whose works included *Der Feurige Elias*, set on and around the narrow-gauge railway that plied between Salzburg and Bad Ischl, and Edmund Eysler, whose sixty works included *Die gold'ne Meisterin*, reputedly Hitler's favourite operetta. The principal operetta librettists of the period also spent their summers in Bad Ischl, lured there by the presence of so many composers and the chance to pitch works at them. They included Alfred Willner, librettist for Puccini's *La rondine* and for ten of Lehár's operettas, Victor Léon, librettist of *Die Lustige Witwe* (*The Merry Widow*), Fritz Löhner-Beda, Alfred Grünwald and Julius Brammer. The close proximity of this talented group of Vienna-based composers and librettists made for a rich interchange of ideas. Much of their work was done in the cafés and bars on the banks of the River Traun, notably the Café Ramsauer and Walther's on the esplanade. Alfred Willner commented: 'Nothing is easier than making an operetta – you just borrow a story and go to a café.' In fact, competition was fierce between librettists and the term '*Operettenbörse*' (operetta stock exchange) was coined to describe the atmosphere in the small Austrian spa town as they vied with each other to come up with suitable texts and sell their ideas to composers.

Of all the figures associated with the silver age of Viennese operetta, it was the acknowledged master of the genre, Franz Lehár, who had the longest and closest connection with Ischl. He first seems to have come in August 1902 and returned for several more summer stays during the 1900s, working among other things on the score of *Die Lustige Witwe*. There is a (possibly apocryphal) story that during his 1903 visit he was driving through Ischl in a one-horse cab when he saw a lady and her young daughter, whom he knew slightly. With his usual courtesy, he offered to drive them back to their lodgings on the outskirts of town and then walk back to his own rented villa nearby. After dropping them off and dismissing the cab, he astonished the pair by suddenly crying out, 'Where is she? Lost! I've left her in the cab,' and dashed back along the road. He had left the half-finished score of *Die Lustige Witwe* in the cab. Maria von Peteani, the young girl who witnessed this rare incident of absent-mindedness on the part of the normally meticulous former regimental bandmaster, went on to become Lehár's principal biographer.

Another young female visitor made a significant impression on Franz Lehár during one of his early summer sojourns in Ischl. The story has it that he first caught sight of Sophie Meth, a Viennese beauty who had entered into a loveless marriage to escape the boredom of her petit bourgeois parental home, from the window of his lodging in Salzburgerstrasse while she was staying in the house opposite. He was captivated by her and made no secret of his feelings. Initially flattered by the attentions of the thirty-six-year-old composer, who was already being pursued by many women, Sophie came to reciprocate his feelings and divorced her first husband to become his lifelong companion, although it was not until 1924 that they married. Lehár stayed in several different lodgings during these early summers in Ischl, of which his favourite was the Rosenvilla, set back from the Esplanade. The pavilion in the garden is said to have been the model for the one in which Camille and Valencienne hide away together in the second act of *Die Lustige Witwe*. Later lodgers in this romantic Biedermeier villa included the composers Emmerich Kálmán, who spent 'three lovely summers amidst the roses', Giacomo Meyerbeer and Julius Bittner, and the librettist Bela Jenbach. At least three major musical scores were largely written in the Rosenvilla, which is now known as the Rosenstöckl and still available for letting over the summer: Meyerbeer's *Dinorah*; Lehár's *Der Graf von Luxemburg*; and Kálmán's *Die Csárdásfürstin*.

In 1912, using the profits from *Die Lustige Witwe*, Lehár bought a substantial villa on the south bank of the River Traun opposite the Hotel Kaiserin Elisabeth. This became his favourite place of work for the rest of his life. The Lehár Villa is now open to the public and preserved exactly as it was when he died there in 1948. The interior has a dark, heavy, rather gloomy feel and the rooms are crammed with antiques, objets d'art and old master paintings. Lehár keenly guarded his privacy when he was composing, usually at night, in his top-floor study furnished with a simple desk and a large Steinway piano. He locked a pair of wrought-iron gates halfway up the staircase so that he could not be disturbed and insisted that his wife sleep in an adjoining house. Alfred Willner, for a long time the composer's favourite librettist, recalled that on one 'sultry, almost suffocating' afternoon in July 1913 he was summoned to Lehár's table at the Café Walther and told that he must come up with a libretto by the following morning. Desperate for a story line, Willner wandered the streets of Bad Ischl and went into the church to pray for inspiration. Then he returned to his rooms, resolving to pass the night in solitary meditation. As he sat alone gazing on the dark mountain peaks, an idea came to him at last: a libretto based on the story of a pair of lovers who climb a peak together to escape the turmoil and frustrations of the world below. The next morning he went round to the composer's villa suggesting that an entire act could be devoted to the two characters alone above the world. Lehár was enthusiastic and thus was born *Endlich Allein* (*Alone at Last*) which he later declared his favourite work. Was this, I wonder, because, like that other song about loneliness in *Der Zarewitsch* (see page 22), it expressed his own introspective yearning as he sat in his solitary spa retreat pouring out his soaring love songs for his near neighbour, Richard Tauber, to sing?

While *Endlich Allein* was playing to packed houses in Vienna in its premiere season in 1914, another of Bad Ischl's most regular summer residents was also feeling his loneliness. Like Franz Lehár, Kaiser Franz Joseph chose to sleep apart from his wife, in his case in a small iron-framed bed in his austere study, which can still be seen by visitors to the Kaiservilla today. It was while sitting in the adjoining study on the afternoon of 28 June that he heard of the assassination of his nephew and heir, Franz Ferdinand, in Sarajevo. His seventy-year-old aide-de-camp took the message on the telephone, which the emperor refused to use, and wrote it down. Stefan Zweig, sitting the following afternoon reading under the chestnut trees in the *Kurpark* at Baden bei Wien, was surprised when the musicians of the *Kurorchester*, playing in the outdoor pavilion in front of the casino, suddenly stopped in mid-bar, packed up their instruments and walked out. He got up and saw that an official communiqué about the assassination had just been posted on the wall. Just under a month later, on 23 July, again in his study in the Kaiservilla, Franz Joseph signed the Austrian ultimatum to Serbia that would trigger the First World War, the event which more than any other brought about the end of the social, political and intellectual conditions in which the European spas flourished.

Spas played an important role in the First World War. Their hotels and bathing establishments were requisitioned as hospitals and convalescent centres for wounded troops. Emperor Karl, who succeeded Franz Joseph in November 1916, established his personal headquarters in a house in the marketplace in Baden bei

Wien and the imperial command subsequently took over a school nearby. It was in Baden two years later that he presided over the dissolution of the Austro-Hungarian Empire and signalled his own withdrawal from any participation in its government. Kaiser Wilhelm II established his personal headquarters in Bad Homburg in 1917, moving in March 1918 to a palatial neo-Norman villa on the outskirts of Spa. A trench was dug in its extensive grounds so that he could be photographed beside it, dressed in a field greycoat and wearing his famous spiked helmet, giving the impression that he was near the front and at the heart of action rather than safe in the secluded garden of a quiet spa town.

The German Supreme Command was already based in Spa in the ironically named Hotel Britannique, a massive and rather forbidding building which is now a boys' school. The final stages of the war were played out there and it was from Spa station that the Kaiser, having announced his abdication, quietly departed at 4.30 a.m. on 10 November 1918 on his way to exile in the Netherlands. His first request when he reached Amerongen Castle was for a 'cup of really hot, strong English tea'.

It was not just emperors who forsook Europe's spas at the end of the war; so did many of the aristocracy, signalling the end of their belle époque. There were other factors in addition to the disruption and social changes caused by the Great War which brought about their demise. The French were following the British in choosing seaside resorts over inland spas and taking themselves off in increasing numbers to the Côte d'Azur, while the Germans were discovering the benefits of bracing mountain air and holidaying in the Alps. But it was not the end of the road for Europe's spas. Thanks to the advent of social democratic policies and national health insurance, they would reinvent themselves in the twentieth century and bounce back as resorts for the masses.

8

THE LAST HUNDRED YEARS

The historic traditional spas of Europe have enjoyed mixed fortunes over the last hundred years. For much of the twentieth century social security and national insurance schemes provided a welcome boost, with middle- and working-class guests replacing their traditional wealthy and aristocratic clientele. This was especially the case in Communist Eastern Europe where spas flourished as popular proletarian holiday resorts to which workers and their families were sent for a couple of weeks a year by trade unions. This process of democratisation changed the culture of spas in several ways, making them less exclusive, more vulgar and less decadent. The end of Communism, together with widespread government spending cuts over recent decades, have meant a diminution in the number of guests paid for through social security and national health insurance schemes, although they still represent a significant presence in the spas of Eastern Europe. Meanwhile, the growth of high-end luxury tourism and the inexorable rise of the wellness industry has brought a new influx of wealthy clients into traditional spas, several of which have successfully rebranded themselves on the basis of their historic charm and appeal. If health, or rather wellness, has become the dominant motif, hedonism and hypochondria have not completely disappeared. Spas have continued to be favourite subjects for novelists and have also caught the attention of film-makers, with *Kurschatten* continuing to exercise a strong fascination in their fictional portrayals along with a deep vein of nostalgia for the luxury, romance and mystery of their bygone golden age.

Although in the short term the First World War provided a new clientele in the substantial number of wounded combatants who frequented them for recuperation and rehabilitation, the war dealt a severe blow to Europe's spas and effectively ended their belle époque. A dramatic indication of their decline is the number of overnight stays by *Kurgäste* in Ragaz, which dropped from 100,000 in 1910 to 48,000 in 1915 and slumped further to 29,000 in 1921. The dismemberment of the German and Austro-Hungarian empires and the impact of the Russian Revolution substantially reduced and impoverished the monarchical and aristocratic classes who had been the spas' most important patrons. Never again would they be the Continent's summer capitals. Instead, they gradually assumed a less flashy and glamorous role, providing cures for the health-conscious middle classes who were more likely to frequent the baths, the *Trinkhalle* and the *Kurpark* than the casino, but were not without their own little indulgences.

A good example of this new kind of spa-goer was the English author Samuel Bensusan who was 'ordered' (a word he emphasised) by his doctor to take a cure in Bad Nauheim in 1922. He took the opportunity of extending his visit to make a more general tour of Germany's *Kurorte* and returned for further travels around them two years later. Initially, he was apprehensive about venturing into Teutonic territory, fearing 'two years' imprisonment in a fortress, if one ventured to walk abroad with a camera; instant death, should one be so foolhardy as to stray upon the grass of a public garden; and a locust-legion of *verbotens* swarming over the most innocent happenings of daily life'. However, these fears proved to be totally unfounded. As well as having a highly successful cure, he found the overall atmosphere of the *Kurorte* delightful and wrote a book about his experiences designed to persuade his fellow countrymen to overcome their understandable post-war prejudices and immerse themselves in 'a world holding out promises not only of renewed health, but of varied interests pursued through tranquil, pleasant days'. *Some German Spas*, published in 1925, enthused about both the natural scenic beauty and the cheerful social ambience of the *Kurorte*. It noted that for every invalid, there might be up to six accompanying family members 'and it is in this happy combination of provision for the sick, who need a physician, and for the healthy, who are seeking a gay time, that the spas have achieved their biggest success' (Bensusan 1925: vii, viii, 20).

Bensusan, who recommended his readers to devote four to six weeks to a cure, followed by an after-cure of two to three weeks in the mountains or by the sea, was a perceptive observer of the ambiguities and contrasts of spa life. In the north German spa of Oeynhausen he was struck by the manifestations of 'tragedy, courage and community in suffering' around the *Kurhaus* 'while the band plays its waltzes of Strauss, Lanner or Waldteufel, or its two-step and three-step by the unknown folk one must try to forgive'. Encounters with war veterans who had suffered physically and mentally and were regaining their health and strength through a prolonged cure prompted him to reflect that 'clearly the spa is good to those who have been stretched too long on the rack of a tough world.' At Bad Ems he was intrigued by how many European and American opera singers took the cure at the end of the season to relieve their strained vocal cords and sinus problems. He noted 'they returned as soon as the war was over, but preserved their incognito, because they did not wish people to know that they were going back to Germany.' In Wiesbaden, he found himself reflecting on the many *Kurgäste* who ventured year after year 'to Spaland in pursuit of a vanishing waist' and undid the good of their morning promenades and sessions in the *Trinkhalle* by spending the afternoons consuming 'chocolate and cakes lavishly overflowing with cream'. Yet despite this backsliding, as he observed the overweight guests taking their morning walks and gradually shedding the cares of everyday life, he felt that even if the pounds were not coming off as much as they might, their cure was nonetheless having its effect: 'heavy steps grow lighter, pale faces win back some of their colour, animation returns to forms that seemed almost too listless to bear the burden of the day' (Bensusan 1925: 26, 27, 57).

Two well-known works by German writers in the mid-1920s give a rather less upbeat picture of the experience of taking a spa cure and dwell more on its tendency to induce melancholy introspection. Thomas Mann's *The Magic Mountain*, published in 1924 and set in a mountain sanatorium on the eve of the First World War, was based on the author's own experience of taking a cure at Bad Gastein as well as on the three weeks he spent in a sanatorium in Davos while his wife was taking a six-month cure there. It reflects the fact that such sanatoria had taken over from spas as the preferred places to go for the treatment of certain conditions, notably tuberculosis which is the disease that Haus Berghof in the novel specialises in curing. Mann powerfully evokes the boredom induced by the long periods of rest and inactivity experienced by the patients and the effects on them of a predictable and prescribed regime in an insulated environment where time ceases to have much meaning. Many become obsessed with the thermometer, or 'the glass cigar' with which they regularly monitor their temperature. One young man, in the sanatorium for eleven months, spends every day lying in bed with it in his mouth and takes no interest in anything else. It is in many ways a terrifying story. The main protagonist, Hans Castorp, first comes to Haus Berghof as a healthy young man to visit his tubercular cousin but falls sick and ends up spending seven years as an in-patient, becoming deeply institutionalised and introspective. The novel's message, according to Mann, is that illness and death provide the necessary passage to knowledge, health and life.

Hermann Hesse described his *Kurgast*, published in 1924, as a 'tolerably candid' account of a cure he had taken the previous year in Baden bei Zürich to seek relief from gout and sciatica. It paints a vivid picture of the introversion and boredom experienced by the spa guest, the irritation provoked by other guests and the obsession that often develops with trivial matters. Stepping off the train, the author is delighted to discover that other *Kurgäste* are in a considerably

worse state and in greater pain than he is. He is somewhat put out
at his initial medical consultation when the doctor, having found
his blood pressure and heart rate to be quite normal, suggests that
his pains might be partly 'psychic' in origin. He insists that they are
genuine and is very relieved when the doctor gives him a lengthy
list of prescriptions for treatments. However, this initial elation soon
gives way to intense annoyance with the noisy Dutchman in the
hotel room next to his own. Increasingly he feels that he is losing
his moral compass in the corrupting atmosphere of what he calls
the 'shadow side' of the spa as he succumbs to its many distractions,
especially gluttony, drinking and gambling. He has his own *Kurschatten*
experience, being briefly captivated by a very pretty young lady
whom he is prepared to forgive when she names as her favourite
books 'several bad works of light fiction' but not when one evening
she sits down at the piano and slaughters a charming eighteenth-
century minuet. Overall, he experiences an intense self-obsessive
egotism. After falling into a state of deep melancholy and distress,
he eventually achieves a sense of peace and liberation but realises
that this has nothing to do with Baden or the cure but rather his
acceptance of divine grace and forgiveness. Despite this somewhat
negative experience, Hesse returned regularly to Baden bei Zürich
for more than twenty-five years, always staying in the same hotel and
finding its atmosphere very conducive to writing novels and poems.

Partly in response to the rise of the Alpine sanatoria, those spas
which were situated in mountainous regions often fared rather
better in the 1920s than the ones in more low-lying areas like Baden-
Baden and Marienbad. As well as their thermal waters, they could
offer healthy mountain air, serious walking in the summer and the
increasingly popular sport of skiing in the winter. Bad Gastein was
one that especially flourished in this period, attracting an eclectic
clientele of regulars including Sigmund Freud, who sat in the radon
gas galleries hoping to mitigate the effects of his six cigars a day, King
Ferdinand of Bulgaria, who spent the evenings driving his Bentley
into the nearby mountains and shooting the deer transfixed by its

headlights, King Faisal of Iraq, and three Indian maharajahs. They all stayed at the sumptuous and massive Grand Hôtel de l'Europe, opened in 1909 with ten floors and its own casino.

Although it was a pale imitation of what the Alpine spas provided for their cavorting kings, the tiny mid-Welsh spa of Llandrindod Wells, which we last encountered building a hall for daily prayer meetings, did its bit to cast off its puritanical pall and take on a rather racier air in keeping with the spirit of the roaring twenties. It was from the Gwalia Hotel there that Frances Stevenson penned love letters to the sixty-one-year-old David Lloyd George in August 1925, telling him: 'I want your lips today, cariad. I have been thinking of their sweetness and their thrillingness, and of course that leads me to think of other things.' Reflecting that the hotel was full of men over sixty, she assured him that 'I would back you for naughtiness against any man of any age ... The old men here may be bald and rheumatic and perfectly virtuous but there is an old man I know in North Wales who is none of these things.' According to local histories, a special external staircase was constructed at the rear of another Llandindrod Wells hotel so that a fellow amorous Welshman, the 2nd Viscount Tredegar, could discreetly reach his private suite.

Perhaps the most dramatic and certainly the most publicised event to take place in a British spa in the 1920s combined mystery, hidden identity and exposure of adulterous betrayal. On 3 December 1926 the crime novelist Agatha Christie disappeared from her home in Surrey. The discovery of her car found perched precariously over the edge of a chalk cliff overlooking a nearby lake led to a nationwide search which involved over 1,000 police officers, troops of Boy Scouts, packs of bloodhounds and numerous members of the public. For the first time ever in a search for a missing person aeroplanes were deployed, while Arthur Conan Doyle, as an acknowledged expert on psychic forces, was brought in to consult the spirit world on her whereabouts. Eleven days after her disappearance she was recognised by the banjo player of the Swan Hydropathic Hotel in Harrogate where she had been staying incognito, having checked in using the surname of her husband's mistress, and enjoying bridge, billiards, dancing and playing the piano among her fellow unsuspecting cure guests. Two doctors certified that she was suffering from amnesia and in one of her very rare comments on the episode, she claimed to have been wandering around in a dream and to have found herself in Harrogate 'as a well-contented and happy woman who believed she had just come from South Africa'. It is now thought more likely that she plotted the entire stunt herself to humiliate her husband and his lover, about whom she had recently learned. It certainly did no harm to her reputation. The nationwide publicity greatly bolstered her fame and contributed to her becoming the world's bestselling novelist with global sales of well over two billion. If it was, indeed, planned, it was surely no coincidence that she chose a spa town in which to stage this dramatic happening which had all the ingredients of one of her own whodunnits. Christie was an enthusiast for thermal medicine and a frequent visitor to Spa, which she made the birthplace of her most famous fictional creation, the detective Hercule Poirot. A plaque in the lobby of what is now called the Old Swan Hotel in Harrogate recalls this bizarre event in the history of a town more usually associated with teacakes, toffee and floral gardens.

It was unusual for spas to be the scenes of such sensational drama and action in this period. More often they were renowned for their dull respectability. This aspect was caught by another famous British thriller writer, John Buchan, in his 1935 story *The House of the Four Winds*, when Alison Westwater describes Unnutz, the fictional Central European *Kurort* where she is stuck with her father, Lord Rhynns, who is taking a cure for neuritis: 'It's a ghastly place which has invented a regime for the idle middle classes of six nations. I do the same things and make the same remarks and wear the same clothes every day at the proper hour. I'm a marionette and so are the other people – quite nice they are, and well mannered, and friendly, but as dead as salted herrings' (Buchan 1993: 45).

The Great Depression of the late 1920s and early 1930s hit European spas hard. In an effort to curb its effects, several invested in new facilities. In Baden bei Wien a vast outdoor art deco open-air lido, the Thermal Strandbad, was built in 1926, complete with a beach made of sand brought from the banks of the Danube. The town's first all-year-round casino was opened in 1934, occupying the former *Kurhaus*. German *Kurorte* increasingly promoted their sports facilities alongside the more traditional attractions of health cures and *Kurschatten*. A poster advertising Bad Ems around 1930 somewhat incongruously highlighted golf, tennis and watersports alongside catarrh, asthma and heart complaints and featured a trio of elegantly dressed ladies gazing down on a young golfer (Plate 10).

A more effective antidote to the Depression was provided by the development of socialised medicine and health insurance schemes which brought a new class of patients to spas and compensated for the loss of their old aristocratic clientele. The French *villes d'eaux* instituted a two-class system of *curistes* with those paying their own way enjoying better facilities. In Vichy the baths in the main Thermal Establishment were reserved for first-class (private) patients while second-class patients had their treatments in the cheaper Bains Callou, housed in a daring angular art deco building erected in 1933. In Germany, by the early 1930s 25 per cent of *Kurgäste* were being paid for through social insurance. Not everyone appreciated this development, as is clear from this comment by a participant in the 1927 conference of the Federation of German Spas:

> The whole atmosphere of the spa or health resort will be lowered, particularly by the practice of treating insurants in company homes, so that the well-to-do guest will no longer see the spa as a place where he can not only recover his damaged health but also relax and generally refresh himself — a necessity sought at least once a year. Thus the private paying guests will turn more and more to foreign resorts where the old atmosphere of luxury and elegance has been preserved, and the consequence must follow that German spas would be proletarianised. (Hüfner 1969: 9)

In fact, the growing number of what became known as 'social cures' almost certainly saved several German *Kurorte* from collapse in the rocky two decades which followed the First World War. In Bad Ems, where the first social cure guests arrived in 1923, the overall number of *Kurgäste* tripled through the 1920s. By contrast, Baden-Baden, which retained its more exclusive cachet and snobbishly shunned 'social cure' patients, suffered badly in the general economic downturn of the period, dropping from 85,531 *Kurgäste* in 1922 to 58,033 in 1932.

The fortunes of the German *Kurorte* were boosted through the 1930s by the rise of Hitler and National Socialism. Largely to raise money, gambling was once again allowed. The Baden-Baden casino reopened in 1933, the year that Hitler became chancellor. Spas were promoted as part of the Nazi cult of *Kraft durch Freude* (KdF) or Strength through Joy, with National Socialist propaganda suggesting that 'a stay in a spa or health resort should … help to educate healthy and sick alike for the structuring of the new German Volk.' Natural medicine, which included balneology, became a compulsory discipline for all medical students, who were encouraged to think in terms of more holistic treatments, embracing wind, sun and fresh air as well as mineral water. Social insurance provision was increased and members of KdF groups, those serving in the armed forces, and less well-off German *Volksgenossen* of Aryan descent were offered free or highly subsidised stays in spas. *Kurorte* were harnessed in the Nazi *Lebensborn* project begun in 1935 to increase the birth rate of 'racially pure' Aryan children. Specially selected statuesque blonde women were sent to Bad Homburg to sleep with high-ranking SS officers to help achieve the Nazi dream of a master race. A crippling 1,000-mark tax imposed in 1933 on Germans going abroad for a holiday or cure also helped to fill the beds in the German *Kurorte*. It devastated the neighbouring Austrian spas, especially Bad Gastein, a favourite resort of Germans, where in 1934 the number of *Kurgäste* fell from 6,000 to 200 and the ninety-five staff in the Grand Hôtel de l'Europe looked after just three guests, one of whom was the king of Belgium.

Other measures implemented by the Nazis were not so beneficial for the German *Kurorte*. Price reductions for foreign guests were abolished, enabling spas in other parts of Europe to attract them — Spa enjoyed its highest ever number of overseas visitors (25,000) in 1938. Jews, who had long been among the most loyal, enthusiastic and free-spending *Kurgäste* in the spas of Germany and Central Europe, were made to feel less and less welcome. Their plight is poignantly portrayed in *Badenheim 1939*, a work written in Hebrew in 1978 by the Israeli novelist, Aharon Appelfeld, and partly based on his memories of childhood visits to Central European *Kurorte* with his parents. It is set on the eve of the Second World War in an Austrian spa town frequented primarily by Jewish guests who are largely oblivious to the activities of the Nazi regime, represented by the 'Sanitation Department', which is systematically engaged in preparing for their removal to concentration camps in Poland. Unaware of their fate, but increasingly frenetic in their behaviour and deranged in their mental state, the Jewish *Kurgäste* gorge themselves on heavy pastries and indulge in *Kurschatten*-type infatuations, with one of the spa doctors falling for a visiting schoolgirl. Overshadowing this desperate hedonism is a gathering sense of impending doom.

The effects of Nazi takeover were felt dramatically in Bad Ischl. On the day after the Anschluss of 12 March 1938 the Gestapo visited the house of Fritz Löhner-Beda, librettist of Lehár's *The Land of Smiles* whose many songs included the original German version of 'Yes! We Have No Bananas' (*Ausgerechnet Bananen!*). He was taken away and put on the first transport from Austria to Dachau concentration camp. Shortly afterwards, the square in the town centre was renamed Adolf Hitler Platz, the main street, Pfarrgasse, became Horst-Wessel Strasse, and Kálmánstrasse was renamed as Anton Bruckner Strasse in an attempt to obliterate the memory of the Jewish operetta composer in favour of the Aryan musician who had played the organ for imperial festivals in the town's parish church.

The Second World War inevitably had a major impact on Europe's spas. Many were requisitioned for the treatment of wounded soldiers. Günter Grass recuperated at Marienbad from shrapnel wounds inflicted by a Russian tank while he was fighting with the Waffen-SS. Others were taken over for military use. In Britain, Woodhall Spa became the base for 617 Squadron of the Royal Air Force, better known as the Dambusters. Their presence there is remembered today in photographs and memorabilia in the Petwood Hotel, a mock-Tudor Edwardian spa hotel which served as the officers' quarters and mess. In France, Vichy became the headquarters of the collaborationist government led by Marshal Pétain in 1940, chosen for its large number of grand hotels and thermal establishments which could accommodate the 30,000 civil servants who descended on the town. Pétain's administration brought new kinds of hypocrisy and *Kurschatten* to *la Reine des villes d'eaux*. Outwardly puritanical and pledged to reverse the liberalising decadence which it claimed had sapped the moral fibre of the Third Republic, it was in reality two-faced and corrupt. A contemporary account by the artist Henri Sjöberg describes steamy affairs among the *fonctionnaires* occupying the opulent spa buildings. As in the German and Austrian spas, Jews were deported from the town. This episode in Vichy's history left a shadow and a sense of shame from which it took a long time to recover.

Several spas suffered considerably during and in the immediate aftermath of the war. The Quellenhof Hotel in Bad Ragaz, which had achieved its official Bad status in 1936, closed in 1939 and did not open again until 1957, while Baden bei Zürich's largest hotel, the Grand, was demolished in 1944 because of the dramatic decline in the number of guests coming even to neutral Switzerland. In Karlsbad fewer than 4,000 *Kurgäste* came in 1945, the lowest number ever, and just 5 per cent of the number thirty-five years earlier. Baden bei Wien lost many of its guests during the years between 1944 and 1955 when it served as the headquarters of the Soviet occupying forces in Austria. For some of the German *Kurorte*, by contrast, occupation by Allied forces helped their revival. The French made Baden-Baden the headquarters of their military occupation zone in

Germany and turned it into a 'little Vichy' by importing French food and prostitutes. A contemporary account from 1945 enthused that '800 colonels are enjoying casino living'. The Americans improved the fortunes of several of the *Kurorte* in their zone of occupation, reopening the casinos in Bad Homburg and Wiesbaden. It took some time for the grand hotels to be cleared from their wartime role as hospitals but by the early 1950s they were open and ready to receive visitors again. In both East and West Germany national health insurance enabled all citizens to spend a subsidised stay at an accredited *Kurort* on the recommendation of a doctor, which was not difficult to obtain. The Austrian spas also bounced back relatively quickly after the war. Thomas Mann had a particularly successful and satisfactory stay at Bad Gastein in the summer of 1951. Not only did the baths there alleviate his arthritis but they also helped the seventy-six-year-old to experience morning erections and to be able to masturbate for the first time in many years. The cure inspired him to resume work on a novel which he had begun forty years earlier but never managed to complete. *Bekenntnisse des Hochstaplers Felix Krull* (published in English as *Confessions of Felix Krull, Confidence Man*) has two scenes set in German *Kurorte*. In the first, eight-year-old Felix, spending several weeks with his family in Bad Schwalbach where his father is taking mud baths to alleviate gout, delights in the spa's tranquil, well-regulated atmosphere and is especially captivated by the daily *Kurorchester* concerts under the direction of its gipsy-like leader. His father buys him a small violin so he can join a Sunday afternoon performance of a Hungarian dance, delighting the fellow *Kurgäste*, who treat him to chocolates and cream puffs at the local confectioner's. The second scene is set in Wiesbaden where, at the age of fourteen, Felix makes his first visit to the theatre and visits the dressing room of the star singer.

It was perhaps just as well that the area of Germany under British occupation after 1945 did not include any of the most famous and fashionable German *Kurorte*. They would not have received much tender loving care from their new masters, who had long ago forsaken spas for the seaside and remained generally sceptical about the supposed benefits of water-based cures. In Britain, the twentieth century saw the progressive closure of those spas that had survived the stampede to the sea. At the end of the First World War there were still nineteen British spas offering treatments using mineral water. By the end of the Second World War the number had shrunk to six. They were incorporated into the new National Health Service when it was created in 1948, with all treatments being offered free, a move which effectively killed off the chances of retaining any private spa guests. For a time it looked as though, as on the Continent, albeit on a smaller scale, the new era of socialised medicine might usher in a boom time for British spas. A report published in 1951 by the British Medical Association, *The Spa in Medical Practice*, sought to promote greater appreciation of their therapeutic potential among doctors. It pointed out that in Britain, unlike most other European countries, medical students received little or no instruction in balneology and other spa treatments and that, as a result, many general practitioners and specialists were unaware of the benefits that some of their patients could derive from them. It recommended that doctors should consider prescribing courses of spa treatment of between three and four weeks for patients with chronic rheumatic diseases and metabolic disorders, certain types of cardiovascular disease, infections of the urinary tract, pelvic conditions in women and disorders of the nervous system. Welcoming the growing emphasis in the medical profession on health rather than disease, and acknowledging the importance of the psychological influence of the spa environment, the report particularly commended the use of spas for rehabilitation and convalescence. It also noted the significant change that had taken place in their clientele: 'There are now fewer wealthy patients and more patients from the lower income groups. Patients nowadays require more modest accommodation and less expensive forms of diversion and recreation, and most of them will come to a spa as National Health Service patients' (BMA 1951: 17).

There was initially a reasonable take-up for these new simpler and less luxurious forms of spa cure. During the 1950s and early 1960s over 250,000 patients annually were receiving treatments at NHS spas, referred by consultants primarily in the areas of rheumatology and orthopaedics. However, pressure on regional health authorities to save money, combined with continuing scepticism on the part of the medical profession, led to the remaining NHS spa facilities being starved of resources and gradually closed. There were some attempts to reverse this trend and secure a brighter future for Britain's spas. A study commissioned by the British Tourist Authority in 1975 recommended making them more attractive by broadening the spectrum of the therapies they offered to include Turkish baths, mud baths, brine baths and inhalations, removing their 'excessively clinical atmosphere' and replacing it 'with a more social ambience'. The problem was that by this time spas in Britain had become oases of political and social conservatism, the chosen abodes of peppery retired colonels and demure elderly ladies congregating in tea shops to mutter about the declining state of the country's morals. Their image was epitomised by the phrase 'Disgusted of Tunbridge Wells' which seems originally to have been coined by local journalists there to sum up the mood of most of the letters received from readers. It was taken up by *Private Eye*, the satirical magazine founded in 1961, and chosen in 1978 as the title for the new BBC Radio 4 programme airing listeners' complaints about programmes, renamed *Feedback* the following year. This was hardly an atmosphere conducive to rebranding Britain's spas with casinos, lap dancing, nightclubs or whatever else might be needed to give them 'a more social ambience'.

I spent my teenage years close to Tunbridge Wells and it was its combination of mysterious bubbling mineral springs, faded elegance and hidden goings-on behind the net curtains of the solid villas that kindled my lifelong fascination with spas. I loved watching the Dipper scoop out cupfuls of the blood-red chalybeate water from her station at one end of the Pantiles and sitting in Binns Restaurant at the other end with my best schoolfriend, trying to shock the elderly blue-rinse brigade with our loud expressions of radical politics. What I did not know then and only discovered recently was that the building which housed Binns has its own *Kurschatten* in the form of a forlorn matronly figure dressed in a long grey dress who haunts the place and can occasionally be seen gazing out of a window on the first floor. There are various suggestions as to who 'the grey lady' might be: a forlorn bride who had been jilted; an assistant in the fashionable milliners' shop watching out for customers; or possibly the madam of the brothel that had occupied the premises in the 1700s, either attempting to lure punters or looking out for one of her girls who had wandered off with a client. She seems to have appeared rather more often since the days when I frequented Tunbridge Wells in the 1960s. At least five sightings of her, always dressed the same and sitting in the same position, were reported in the 1990s. I like to think that she is actually the ghost of a 1960s Tunbridge Wells matron outraged at the teatime chatter of me and my friend and looking out in case we return. Alas, the building which she haunts is no longer a genteel tea room but a Mediterranean restaurant with 'The Grey Lady Music Lounge' above it featuring live jazz and blues. In that respect, as in others, Tunbridge Wells has moved with the times and thrown off its previous dowdy and demure image.

By the time my own interest in spas began in the mid-1960s, there were few working ones left in Britain. Buxton's baths were closed in 1966 and the Royal Baths in Harrogate three years later. In 1976, the NHS stopped funding medical treatments using the thermal waters in Bath and two years later the discovery of a lethal organism led to the closure of all the baths there. Treatments stopped at Woodhall Spa in 1983 and the last NHS facility using thermal mineral water, the physiotherapy and hydrotherapy departments at the Royal Pump Room in Leamington Spa, finally closed in 1997. For some time after their closure, these former baths and pump rooms exuded an aura of decay and neglect, providing a sad testament to the final ending of the once pioneering British love affair with spas. More recently, however, several have been renovated and found new uses. Harrogate's Turkish baths were restored and reopened in 2004, its old Royal Baths now house a Chinese restaurant and its former pump room is a museum. The old pump room at Leamington has also been turned into a museum and art gallery and Buxton's former natural baths house a shopping arcade. After decades of neglect and a seemingly endless period of construction work, restoration of the Georgian Crescent at the heart of Buxton is due to be completed in 2020, with the opening of a new spa hotel using the thermal waters and refurbished assembly rooms.

America's best-known and most European spa went through a similar process of decline over the same period. Saratoga Springs had already lost all of its grand hotels by 1960, thanks to the departure of its rich clientele and a growing disenchantment with hydrotherapy and its benefits. The Washington Baths closed in 1978, reopening in 1986 as a National Museum of Dance. The Lincoln Baths limped on half-empty before they, too, were closed in 2005, leaving only some of the cubicles in the Roosevelt Bath House remaining open for massages and baths. When I visited that year, the whole place had a gloomy deserted feel, the Gideon Putnam Hotel almost empty in the middle of the Spa State Park with its sombre 1930s neoclassical buildings set among tall, dark, brooding pine trees. There has been some revival since but the place is still a shadow of what it was in its heyday.

In contrast to the sorry story of what happened in Britain and the United States, many Continental spas continued to prosper through the second half of the twentieth century. In Germany's case this was in large part thanks to an increasing number of social cures. Their impact can be clearly seen in statistics relating to Bad Ems. In 1949 for the first time it welcomed more *Kurgäste* funded out of social insurance than paying privately. By 1953 it had more *Kurgäste* than at any previous time (12,271) and four years later the number had reached 16,359, its highest total ever.

Not everyone was happy about the impact that social cures were having, not just on the ambience of *Kurorte* but also in medical terms. In an article published in 1965 Dr Schretzenmayr, a well-regarded practitioner in internal medicine, suggested that they encouraged the besetting spa disease of hypochondria and acted against the interests of the really ill. He expressed misgivings about the selection procedures for patients, complaining that many of his sick patients were being turned away from clinics because no beds were available while 'the vast majority of cure "patients", hypochondriacs, healthy, not-totally healthy or not-yet-ill, loll about in social feather beds.' He was also highly critical of the insurance companies' policy of building cure clinics in attractive, out-of-the-way spas rather than in places of real need: 'If the social insurance [bodies] have money to spare for a clinic then surely it should not be built in *Klein-Kleckersdorf an der Knatter* but rather at the centres of need and for the sick!' (Schretzenmayr 1965: 134–5).

Such criticisms were few and far between, however, and in general throughout the 1960s and 1970s the growth of *Kurorte* was welcomed and social cures were enthusiastically promoted by the medical establishment. In 1972 the Federation of German Spas produced a new more comprehensive definition of the spa cure which combined the growing interest in alternative medicine with an acknowledgement that more conventional therapies, including drugs, could also play a role:

A cure is a remedial process characterised by the repeated application of preponderantly natural remedies according to a plan prescribed by a doctor and which entails a change of surroundings and environment. Treatment at a spa consists of a general therapy, which is systematically structured and which, besides natural remedies, also uses physical medicine, locomotive therapy, diet, psychotherapy and also treatment with drugs, all tailored to individual needs. (Deutscher Bäderverband 1972: 33)

Such a cure was to be achieved through an 'ordering of the forces of the organism' involving

> relief from work and the regulated world of the work place; the harmonisation of daily rhythms consisting of changes between periods of concentration, relaxation, nutritional intake and sleep; a healthy diet; additional exercise or rest to compensate for the one-sided demands of everyday life; leisure as a precondition for the innermost order of one's life; the elimination of harmful factors in the climate and the avoidance or restriction of such 'pleasures' as cigarettes, alcohol, coffee, sweets etc. (Deutscher Bäderverband 1972: 46–7)

The Spa Federation commended a specific range of therapies, including balneotherapy in its various forms (bathing and drinking cures), climatic therapy, including sun and fresh air cures, diet, supplementary physical therapies involving movement and exercise, various forms of gymnastics, physiotherapy and sports, hydro- and thermotherapy, electrotherapy, light and radiology treatment, inhalation therapy, massages and specific Kneipp and Priessnitz treatments.

Research undertaken at this time pointed to the effectiveness of such spa cures. In 1967 Dr Wannenwetsch, a medical practitioner attached to the Regional Insurance Department in Swabia, published a cost–benefit analysis of the benefits of spa treatments by comparing the periods of sick leave taken by patients before and after taking a cure. He found that whereas 62 per cent of patients had taken a period of sick leave in the year prior to their cure, only 31 per cent did so in the year following it. In an overall study of 7,000 patients over ten years, he concluded that the number of days lost at work was reduced by 63.5 per cent because of the cures they had taken. Other studies focused on asking patients how they themselves felt. A survey undertaken by academics in the University of Ulm in 1973 asked *Kurgäste* how they felt when starting their treatments; 86 per cent replied 'unwell, unsure, tired, nervous or lonely'. At the end of their three-week cures, when asked the same question, only 43 per cent still described their condition in those terms, while 57 per cent reported feeling 'happy' or 'well'.

Other aspects of the *Kur* were also subjected to academic analysis, not least the ubiquitous *Kurschatten*. In his critical 1965 article, Dr Schretzenmayr described the sexual behaviour of cure guests as 'excessive' and recommended that there should always be an accompanying member of the family to discourage rash affairs and liaisons. A survey conducted in 1979 among medical practitioners across German *Kurorte* similarly noted that 'the presence of a partner could deal with the *Kurschatten* problem which was taken very seriously by some doctors.' It quoted a newspaper article written by a journalist who joined a group of women undertaking a cure and reported that within a few days of it starting, 'most had already found themselves *Kurschatten* from the neighbouring clinic.' However, medical opinion was not unanimous on this topic. In the course of her research during the 1980s on Bad Ems, Jackie Bennett-Ruete was told by one doctor that the success rate of cures was significantly enhanced by patients' encounters with *Kurschatten*, which he regarded as 'of considerable therapeutic value' (Bennett-Ruete 1987: 326).

The persistence of *Kurschatten* in various forms in other Continental spas is evident from fictional evocations of spa life in the mid-twentieth century in three notable films. *The Great Sinner*, made in 1949 and starring Gregory Peck and Ava Gardner, is a story of fatal addiction to the roulette tables filmed in Wiesbaden and based on Dostoyevsky's *The Gambler*. Alain Resnais' *L'Année dernière à Marienbad* (*Last Year at Marienbad*) (1961), with a screenplay by Alain Robbe-Grillet, conveys the dreamlike, fluid, fantasy character of the *Kurort* even though it was actually filmed at castles around Munich because the communist authorities in Czechoslovakia felt it was too decadent and would not give permission for it to be made in Marienbad. It is about an unnamed man who wanders the halls and passageways of 'an enormous, luxurious, baroque, lugubrious hotel, where corridors succeed endless corridors' in search of a woman with whom he claims to have had a passionate affair there the previous year. She insists that they have never met, raising the question of whether he is fantasising or dreaming. Robbe-Grillet has said that the film deals with a reality which the hero creates out of his own vision and his own mind. It all seems to be going on inside his head, providing, perhaps, the ultimate *Kurschatten*. There are other spa shadows in the film – a haunting melancholy, a yearning and longing, and a world filled with memories and poised between reality and fantasy, all evoked by the endless eerily silent deserted corridors, seeming to belong to another century, through which the man wanders. The third spa film from this period, Federico Fellini's *8½* (1963), based on the director's own experience of taking a cure at the Tuscan spa of Chianciano Terme, centres around Guido Anselmi, an Italian film director who has shut himself up in a spa to try to recover from creative block. While there, he is visited by both his mistress and his wife and experiences fantasies involving prostitutes and being bathed and powdered by a harem of lithe women. Like *L'Année dernière à Marienbad* it is essentially about a man retreating into his private thoughts and fantasies, many of which are in the form of *Kurschatten*, with the spa setting contributing to the air of unreality, desperation and decadence.

The *Kurschatten* theme is also prominent in two novels set in spas in this period. Bruce Chatwin's *Utz* describes a visit to Vichy by Kaspar Utz, a lonely, introverted Czech porcelain collector in 1952. To escape the oppressive atmosphere of Communist Prague, he persuades his doctor to diagnose a malfunctioning liver as the cause of his persistent depression and prescribe a month in the French spa. To his surprise, given the reputation of more accessible Czech spas like Marienbad and Karlsbad for treating this condition, the authorities let him go, although his copy of Thomas Mann's *The Magic Mountain* is confiscated by Czech customs officers as he crosses the border. This was a time when Vichy was undergoing a renaissance, attracting a large number of guests from Algeria and a glittering array of celebrity *curistes* including Prince Rainier of Monaco. The town boasted thirteen cinemas, eight dance halls and three theatres. The novel, written in 1987 when Chatwin was suffering from AIDS, gives little sense of this glamour and gaiety. Utz finds most aspects of his cure unpleasant; the mud baths, the pressure showers, his sessions with a clearly psychologically disturbed masseur and '*les instruments de torture*' inflicted on him by the severe disciplinarian ladies who staff the Grand Établissement Thermal. He feels bored, becoming worried that he is being stalked by solitary men and depressed by the number of severely wounded servicemen and the drawn, dyspeptic faces of his fellow *curistes* who are clearly finding the experience as miserable as he is.

Having imbibed the idea from reading Russian novels that 'a spa-town was a place where the unexpected invariably happened', Utz has come determined to find romance in Vichy, as his parents did when they met in Marienbad. Convinced that one of the many solitary female *curistes* will almost literally fall into his arms without him having to pursue her, he eyes up various possibilities before settling on a tall lithe woman in tennis whites whom he sees in the hotel lobby. He follows her as she walks her dog along the Allier but she shuns his attempts at conversation and turns the other way when he passes her table at dinner that evening. The following morning he sees her leave the hotel with a handsome man in a sports car. Dejected and depressed, he cuts short his cure and returns to Prague.

W. G. Sebald's *Austerlitz* includes a lengthy passage about a stay in Marienbad in 1972 by the novel's enigmatic and eponymous central figure. He has come there in an attempt to rid himself of an insidious illness of 'self-inflicted isolation'. On a previous visit in 1938, when he was just four, the Czech spa had radiated a sense of peacefulness but now he finds it a disturbing and haunted place, full of mirrors and ghosts. On a walk through the deserted town to the fountain colonnade Austerlitz keeps feeling as if someone else is walking beside him, or as if something is brushing against him. The decrepit state of the once magnificent buildings, with their broken gutters, boarded-up windows and crumbling plaster, reflects and enhances his own sense of melancholy. He feels that the buildings know something ominous about him and point to his acute loneliness. Overall, the atmosphere of the spa evokes hidden memories, some happy but others deeply unsettling.

These portrayals of spas as haunted places of memories and dreams, not quite of this world, reflected the growth of a more general impression which wrapped them in nostalgia and saw them as quaint survivors from an earlier age. Perhaps this view gained ground partly because one of their basic functions and selling points was being challenged by new technological developments and inventions. In 1948 Candido Jacuzzi, one of seven brothers who had emigrated from Italy to California at the beginning of the twentieth century and set up a family business making aircraft propellers and water pumps, developed a submersible bath tub pump so that his son, who had rheumatoid arthritis, could have soothing whirlpool treatments at home. Initially manufactured and sold simply as a therapeutic aid, 'The Roman', as it was originally called, provided an artificially induced version of the bubbling thermal waters found in Aquae Sulis and other ancient spas. Renamed the Jacuzzi, it was launched on the wider market in 1968 as the world's first self-contained, fully integrated whirlpool bath. With its Roman inspiration and therapeutic origins locating it in historic spa culture, the Jacuzzi was perfectly timed to hit the dawning of the Age of Aquarius and, creating its own new ritual around the hot tub, helped to make 1970s California a byword for self-indulgent decadence and a haven for hedonism. Although its heartland remained the United States, where 400,000 hot tubs are now sold every year, it spread to Europe and beyond. Marketed as 'family spas', the hot tubs, saunas and thermal whirlpool baths manufactured by Jacuzzi and other companies allowed people to have a spa experience in their own home. They were installed in hotels and in the leisure clubs and gyms which mushroomed from the late 1980s as part of the new fitness cult. With the proliferation of these ultra-modern, utilitarian gadgets, which took the name 'spa' and brought the experience of bathing in bubbling hot water to the home and the high street, it was not surprising that the appeal of the traditional spas came to lie more in their history, culture, distinctive atmosphere and medical expertise and that they increasingly sold themselves on the basis of these features.

Evidence of this approach comes from the promotional material produced by leading European spas in the early 1980s which combined bold medical claims backed by detailed research findings with reminders of their extensive cultural and recreational facilities. A glossy brochure produced by La Société des Sciences Médicales de Vichy in 1980 trumpeted the benefits of both drinking and bathing cures for those with digestive and metabolic disorders, rheumatism and the after-effects of osteoarticular trauma. Complex graphs tracked the effects of post-operative ingestion of Vichy water on levels of gastric ulceration among rats and the impact of cures on a range of disorders including migraine, dyspepsia, viral hepatitis and 'hypochondriac pain'. *Curistes* were informed that the daily prescribed dose of water rarely exceeded 350 to 400 grammes (0.35 to 0.4 litres, or around half a pint), compared to several litres in the past. They were also warned to expect several thermal crises during a typical twenty-one-day cure but reassured that these had no disturbing significance and simply showed the 'in-depth' effects of the water. Although the overall tone was scientific and clinical, the brochure also alluded to the entertainment on offer to those who chose to take a cure in Vichy, with its eleven cinemas, four theatres, two casinos, two libraries, two bridge clubs and two bullfights a year.

A similar brochure produced by the Spa Directorate at Bad Gastein, entitled *A Hot Spring in the Doctor's Service*, was even more packed with detailed research findings and cited numerous scientific studies to show the efficacy of the radon-rich waters. Photographs showed the beneficial effects of subcutaneous injections of Gastein thermal water on the seminal vesicles of young, sexually mature and elderly mice and on the uteruses of guinea pigs, while a graph showed the markedly increased level of urine excretion achieved after drinking the thermal water as against ordinary tap water. This impressive accumulated evidence would seem to point to the spa being especially geared to treating the impotent, the infertile and the incontinent. However, the brochure focused largely on the benefits of the 'healing radon' to those suffering from rheumatism while also quoting a doctor's verdict in 1576 that the water 'even came to the aid of loose teeth' as testament to its benefits for sufferers from periodontal disease. Those contemplating a cure in Bad Gastein were left in no doubt that health came before hedonism, being reminded: 'a cure is *not a holiday* but a therapeutic treatment, which can *only be effective* if you and your body co-operate.' But they were also promised comfortable accommodation ranging from luxury hotels to inexpensive country pensions, Austria's largest winter sports centre, hunting, fishing, promenades and rambles in 'an unbounded *Kurpark*' as well as concerts, theatre, cabaret and lectures.

More wide-ranging philosophical reflections on the nature and future of spas feature in *Swiss Spas Today* published by the Swiss Spas Collective in Bad Ragaz in 1981. The small booklet contained a fascinating apologia for spa medicine by Dr J. C. Terrier, a rheumatologist long based in Baden bei Zürich who died in 1992. Arguing that both the psychological aspects of spa therapies, and the psychosomatic nature of many of the conditions which led people to try them, had tended to devalue their status in serious medicine, he suggested that they could, in fact, bring enhanced medical benefits, not least through the unique position of the spa physician who, unlike the busy general practitioner, is

a person to whom you can open yourself, expose your sores, and trust your intimate problems under a two-fold guarantee: the first being that he will give your story his full attention without being sparing of his time; the second being that you will not see him again later in daily life. The spa physician will be your friend and adviser during the three weeks of your stay. He will listen and listen and listen. But then, he will vanish from your life. (Terrier 1981: 28)

Terrier went on to list the key positive influences provided by a spa cure and not found in other forms of medical treatment. They included the old-fashioned architecture and ambience 'which brings one back to the good old times, when everything was easier, quieter, and more dignified', the diversions and distractions, the opportunity to discuss one's complaints with fellow sufferers and the ritual inherent in the sequence of baths and treatments, fixed meal times and prescribed periods of rest, enabling life to fall into a set rhythm and inner tensions to be appeased. He even commended the long periods of ennui and killing time as an antidote to the prevailing restlessness of the modern age: 'Doing nothing may have sometimes a therapeutic value. It must be learned, and can best be learned in a spa.' He also waxed positively lyrical when writing about the spring or source at the heart of every spa:

At the risk of sounding mystic, romantic and unscientific, I dare to state that the water of the spring does not carry only the chemical and physical agents which are objectively traceable. On the subconscious level, it is also loaded with a meaning and a message, to which every man will more or less respond, and to which each age of mankind has responded in the past.

It recalls the eternal resurgence and rebirth of life: always new and always the same, always flowing and always generous. The springs are a symbol of all beginnings. They bring the thoughts of man back to its natural origin. And the return to the sources is often the first step towards a renewal (Terrier 1981: 33).

This unostentatious and rather serious Swiss publication presented a convincing case for the future of spas through embracing the psychosomatic basis of many disorders and the psychological aspects of their cures in the context of modern concerns about imperfect work–life balance, stress and burnout. It is one of the earliest documents that I have seen emphasising wellness, the concept that now dominates the whole spa industry. In a contribution on the future of spas, Peter Kasper, President of the Swiss Spas Association, wrote: 'guests cannot be induced to take a course of preventive treatment at a spa by talking about sickness and cures', rather 'they must be sold health.' He went on to suggest that spas should not be compared with hospitals 'full of peevish patients' but should rather see themselves as 'health centres with diversified facilities for sport and cultural activities, games and recreation, as places for a more elevated lifestyle' (Kasper 1981: 67).

Another more official document from 1983, published by the European Regional Office of the World Health Organisation (WHO), indicates a dawning realisation of the potential role of spas in the healthcare of an increasingly ageing population. A report by a working party set up to assess the contribution of balneotherapy to the healthcare of the elderly concluded that the therapeutic use of thermal waters could have an important role to play in the maintenance of health and the reduction of certain disabilities in later life. It recommended further research in this area and the inclusion of balneotherapy in WHO programmes. Although there has been less follow-up of these recommendations than there might have been, many spas have found themselves catering for a largely elderly clientele and have developed exercise and fitness regimes to combat the effects of ageing.

For the most part, the traditional Continental European spas prospered in this period, with several achieving their highest ever visitor numbers in the early 1980s. In Germany in 1980 around six million people took a spa cure, triple the number twenty-five years earlier, and half of all tourist nights were spent in the country's more than 300 officially recognised *Kurorte*. Bad Ragaz achieved its highest ever number of *Kurgäste* in 1981, with a total of 390,770 overnight stays, more than triple the total twenty years earlier. Spas in the communist countries of Eastern Europe were particularly flourishing. By the mid-1980s more than five times as many Yugoslavs, Czechs and Hungarians were taking an annual cure as the Germans and French combined. Equipped with somewhat soulless sanatoria and medical facilities, the traditional *Kurorte* in the eastern part of the former Austro-Hungarian Empire became state-subsidised resorts for those working in the new collectivised factories and farms who were sent by their trade union or through social insurance schemes for annual two- or three-week rest cures. Organised like holiday camps, the communist spas had a strongly collective and proletarian ethos, their once elegant hotel dining rooms being turned into workers' canteens and their ballrooms and theatres becoming dance halls and cinemas.

These developments were evident when I toured the spas of Yugoslavia and Czechoslovakia in the mid-1980s. I have already shared my impressions of the sulphurous spring in Ilidža on the outskirts of Sarajevo (see page 28). In the nearby spa of Kiseljak, the Hotel Dalmacija displayed a notice in English proudly proclaiming 'We are engaging in sanitary tourism.' It specialised in treating those with diabetes, ulcers and other intestinal problems by getting them to drink copious quantities of the local mineral water which is rich in magnesium, thallium and calcium. At first sight, it did not look very inviting. Through a locked glass door marked 'Terapija', all I could see was a dingy hall containing two broken chairs and an empty tub from which two cracked pipes protruded. It turned out that all the treatments were carried out in the basement. Dr Vedad Seremet, one of six doctors working in the hotel, who like all Yugoslav medics had spent six months of his training studying the therapeutic applications of mineral waters, proudly took me round his subterranean domain, every so often grabbing my notebook to draw anatomical diagrams showing the actions of the mineral-rich waters on the cell walls of ulcerated stomachs and thrusting into my hand a blue porcelain flask of the scalding hot water which was so highly mineralised that it formed white encrusted deposits.

When I expressed reservations about drinking it, he said that he was planning to add perfume to give the water a less unpleasant taste and smell but assured me that the hotel guests downed it daily in its natural state without any ill effects. The dark red-tiled treatment rooms housed large baths for underwater massage and what looked alarmingly like an electric chair, to which were attached basins for bathing the arms and legs. Even more alarming were what Dr Seremet delicately called 'bath rooms without water for the whole body' in which patients sat naked while the natural gas, found in the same underground caverns as the mineral water, was pumped in around them. Upstairs, while chain-smoking and drinking small cups of thick Turkish coffee, he told me that about two-thirds of those taking the waters at Kiseljak were factory workers sent there and paid for by their employers or the state. They stayed either for ten to fifteen days for a general rest, or twenty-one days if they were seeking a cure for a specific illness.

At Rogaška Slatina, a long-established spa north of Zagreb, the English-language brochure recommended drinking, bathing and mud baths for 'all of acute (sharp) sicknesses of the gastrointestinal system, chronic alcoholism and psychiatric patients in the bad condition'. The therapeutic effects of its magnesium-rich waters were first discovered in 1680 when an Austrian count was apparently successfully treated for hardening of the arteries. The long-term effects of his cure could not be measured as he was shortly afterwards beheaded for treason. I joined a crowd gathered in the modern circular drinking hall of the Hotel Donat. It was all I could do to manage more than a few mouthfuls of the tepid Donat water, which tasted like warm Alka-Seltzer, but all around me determined drinkers were draining large glasses of the cloudy, effervescent liquid and coming back for more. Most were purposefully walking round in silence and looking out through plate-glass windows to the courtyard outside where the effervescent water bubbled and surged through a series of cylindrical glass columns, much as it would be through their own intestines.

A similarly serious atmosphere prevailed in Banja Koviljača, eighty-five miles south-west of Belgrade, once one of the most fashionable Balkan spas in the nineteenth century. The elegant summer villas had been turned into sanatoria and nursing homes and the ornamental gardens were full of wheelchairs and people on crutches. Between 1970 and 1998, the thermal establishment here was known as the 'Institute for dissipated and post-traumatic conditions'. There was not much sign of dissipation in any form when I took lunch in solitary silence in the sepulchral dining room of the late nineteenth-century Hotel Podrinje, served by a waiter whose demeanour and countenance was suggestive of a born undertaker's mute. The meal was of a blandness that would cause no disturbance to the most sensitive stomach – a clear, watery soup followed by a minute portion of over-cooked pork floating in a sea of liquidised spinach. Outside, a long line of crippled elderly ladies painfully made their way to a gaudily painted drinking fountain where they filled their cups and bottles. Beyond stretched what had once been the *Kurpark*, now overgrown with crumbling fountains and summer houses and a large *Kursalon*, which still had fine gilded mirrors in its entrance hall but was completely empty apart from a long line of coat hangers suspended on metal rails. A gaunt sanatorium half hidden by trees on the hillside above contributed to the rather eerie Gothic atmosphere. As in all the Yugoslav spas I visited there was little evidence of either hedonism or hypochondria. Rather the overall impression was of genuinely ill patients focused on the serious business of drinking or bathing in the waters in rather grim surroundings suggestive of past glories and faded elegance.

The Czech spas of Marienbad (renamed Mariánské Lázně), Karlsbad (Karlovy Vary) and Franzensbad (Františkovy Lázně) to which I took my long-suffering wife on our honeymoon in 1986 were also primarily focused on the medical side of spa life. The great majority of those staying there were Czechs taking holidays and rest cures paid for by trade unions or the state. There were also significant numbers of Russians and East Germans benefiting from inter-governmental agreements and a sprinkling of Western and Middle Eastern guests, attracted by the low prices and keenly courted, as in Yugoslavia, by a communist government desperate to inject hard foreign currency into the ailing domestic economy. From 1980 several Czech spas started specialising in geriatric medicine and offering anti-ageing treatments. These were heavily dependent on the controversial drug Gerovital rather than on more traditional and natural water-based spa therapies and were targeted at the over-fifties, with a preventative programme for those in their forties.

Karlovy Vary had lost much of its belle-époque charm and appeal and had a distinctly seedy feel. The air was heavily polluted from the nearby petrochemical works and many of the buildings were crumbling and shabby. The springs and bath houses had largely lost their old names and were simply given a number, so that one was directed to Bath House No. 3 or Spring No. 12. In the hotel in which we were staying, prostitutes lined up in the bar every evening. The manager told us that they were there for the Arab guests, who came for the *Mädchen* rather than the cure. We were also told that the spa still had a reputation for amorous liaisons, with locals referring to the many 'colonnade couples' who got together while parading around the drinking halls. The Big Brother influence of Russian Communism was very evident in the spa area where the concrete and glass-walled drinking hall, which enclosed the twelve-foot-high jet of water from Spring No. 1 and the fountains from which to drink its waters at various temperatures, was named after the Soviet cosmonaut Yuri Gagarin. The Grandhotel Pupp had been rebranded as the Hotel Moskva.

Mariánské Lázně presented a less shabby and seedy appearance. The air was much less polluted, the main spa buildings in a better state and rather more appealing diversions and distractions were offered to the morning and afternoon promenaders who thronged the main colonnade drinking the water through the spouts of what looked like inverted teapots to avoid discolouring or damaging their teeth. Several significant improvements were made to the spa area here during the 1970s and 1980s, including the complete reconstruction of the great cast-iron drinking hall, which was renamed the Maxim Gorky colonnade and decorated with rather crude frescoes depicting Soviet cosmonauts, and the refurbishment of the neoclassical Karolina Spring pavilion. The Singing Fountain, a stone- and stainless-steel structure incorporating 250 water jets, synchronised to accompany a programme of recorded music played every two hours from 7 a.m. until 9 p.m., was installed at the end of the colonnade in 1986. Although we were regaled with stories of infidelities and *Kurschatten*-style spa romances, the overall atmosphere seemed to be more innocent and staid than in Karlovy Vary. Perhaps this had something to do with the fact that top of the list of the complaints for which the Mariánské Lázně waters were recommended were 'diseases of the urinary pathways' – hardly a recipe for wild affairs. The side streets were lined with huge cheap hotels and sanatoria packed with well-built middle-aged Czech couples who could be glimpsed through the ground-floor windows in the evening dancing to ballads like '*Volare*' and '*O Sole Mio*' belted out by a singer accompanying himself on a primitive electronic keyboard. *The Times* journalist Jonathan Meades, who visited Mariánské Lázně in 1988, found it full of Kuwaitis, Russians and Hungarians, and gained a similar impression. While noting that 'newly-met couples enjoying freshly-minted flings gambol with ever deserting inhibition till they dare dance *le slow*, cheek to worker's cheek, wiggling a little the way those reprogrammed into youth always will', he concluded that: 'Although people come by themselves – subbed by the state, spouseless, cash-heavy, spruce in new threads, looking for a good time, the prevailing air is one of innocence earnestly indulged. It's all rather like the more sedate sort of British resort a long time ago – Scarborough in the Thirties, say ... It might be Bournemouth' (Meades 1988: 13).

Františkovy Lázně, the third of the great spas of Western Bohemia, had a more elegant and more clinical feel than its two better-known neighbours on our 1986 visit. I had not realised when

I booked a room there for the culmination of our honeymoon that it specialised in the treatment of gynaecological conditions. The (very) small print in the brochure on the table between our twin hospital-style beds in the sanatorium-like residence where we were staying spelled these out in all too graphic terms: 'infertility, disorders of ovarian function, chronic inflammatory diseases of internal genital tract, conditions after operations on internal genitals, disturbances of the menstrual cycle'. Within minutes of our arrival, we were told to report to the *Krankenschwester* and our first evening meal consisted of a minuscule plate of grapes and a few dry biscuits. Thankfully, my wife was not wheeled away during the night for treatment, as I rather feared she might be, and in the morning I was able to establish with reception that we were seeking a holiday rather than medical treatment and for the rest of our brief stay we were able to enjoy the rather calm, classical atmosphere of this underrated spa.

The fall of Communism in Eastern Europe at the end of the 1980s had an initially negative impact on its spas. It severely curbed the lavish subsidised provision of spa holidays for all workers. The break-up of Yugoslavia in 1992 and subsequent violent ethnic conflicts in the Balkans through the 1990s effectively ended the life of several of the region's most prominent spas. Kiseljak suffered particularly in the conflicts, with the Hotel Dalmacija being destroyed, and it has not reopened as a spa since. Ilidža became the headquarters of a NATO-led multinational peacekeeping Stabilisation Force in Bosnia and Herzegovina (SFOR) from 1996 to 2006 with the former thermal hotels being occupied by soldiers. Since then, it has reopened its spa facilities and now boasts a modern Spa Terme Hotel standing in a forty-hectare park. Rogaška Slatina, now in Slovenia, suffered less and has remained a working spa with the Hotel Donat undergoing expensive refurbishment to cash in on the booming modern wellness industry. Banja Koviljača, in Serbia, is also still in business as a spa although the Hotel Podrinje, where I had the watery soup, is permanently closed. Karlovy Vary, Mariánské Lázně and Františkovy Lázně, now in the Czech Republic, took an initial hit after the fall of Communism but have benefited from substantial new investment over recent decades and now attract many foreign guests, especially Germans and Russians, being considerably cheaper than neighbouring German and Austrian spa resorts (see pages 275 and 277–8). The Eastern European countries which formerly espoused communism, notably Czechoslovakia, Poland and Hungary, continue to provide more in the way of subsidised spa cures and holidays than their Western neighbours. They also remain generally more enthusiastic about the therapeutic effects of thermal mineral waters.

Western European spas too experienced a period of quite serious decline from the later 1980s. Most had become heavily dependent on subsidised 'social cures'. In Bad Ems in 1985, for example, only 1,667 *Kurgäste* were paying for their own treatments as against 8,505 funded through social security. This made the considerable reductions in state support for spa cures which began in Germany in the mid-1980s a serious blow. As well as reducing the overall funding for spa treatments, the minimum waiting period between cures was increased to three years and those over fifty-nine were excluded from subsidised rehabilitation programmes. In 1993 the Belgian government stopped reimbursing people for cures, effectively ending spa treatments in Spa which had become largely dependent on state support. Similar economies in France through the 1980s and 1990s led to a dramatic fall in the number of *curistes* coming to the main *villes d'eaux*. Vichy suffered a decline from 140,000 *curistes* in the mid-1960s to less than 20,000 in 2002. Another blow came in the wake of the AIDS epidemic in the late 1980s which led to the closure of several Turkish baths and bath houses associated with homosexual promiscuity. More broadly it unleashed a new puritanism which somewhat tarnished the image of spas.

Against this background, the 1990s were a gloomy decade for Europe's traditional spas. Their historic bath houses, pump rooms, grand hotels and other public buildings were showing signs of neglect with several being closed and boarded up. In so far as they were seen as having a future, it seemed to be as part of the booming heritage industry by cashing in on the growing mood of nostalgia, harking back to their past glories and selling themselves primarily as tourist attractions on the basis of their unique architecture and ambience. This thinking lay behind a tourist route developed in 1998 around seventeen of the *villes d'eaux* in the Auvergne and Massif Central area of France. Similar considerations have underlain two more recent initiatives. The European Historic Thermal Towns Association (EHTTA), founded in 2009 by Acqui Terme, Bath, Salsomaggiore Terme, Spa, Vichy and Ourense in Spain, is now a network of nearly fifty spa towns across seventeen countries committed to preserving and publicising Europe's thermal cultural heritage and promoting travel to spa towns through ventures such as 'The European Route of Historic Thermal Towns', one of the cultural routes launched and certified by the Council of Europe. In 2019 eleven 'Great Spas of Europe' – Spa, Bath, Vichy, Baden bei Wien, Karlovy Vary, Františkovy Lázně, Mariánské Lázně, Baden-Baden, Bad Ems, Bad Kissingen and Montecatini Terme – made a joint bid for UNESCO World Heritage status.

At around the same time as the heritage lobby was waking up to the urgent need to preserve and protect them as valuable and threatened architectural and cultural gems, film directors were finding Europe's crumbling spas evocative locations and backdrops for screenplays treating familiar themes of decadence, hedonism and *Kurschatten*. An early example was the 1973 French film *Belle*, set in Spa, which portrays a passionate affair between an ageing married man and a mysterious young foreign girl who hardly understands a word that he says. The Gellért Baths in Budapest have proved a particularly popular location for films with a strong sexual theme, including *Accumulator 1* (1994) about a man whose sexual energy is drained from him by television; *Cremaster 5* (1997), a tragic love story based around a five-act lyric opera with frequent shots of sexual reproduction (the title refers to the cremaster muscle which is responsible for raising and lowering the male testes in order to regulate their temperature); *Pools of Desire*, originally titled *Viz* (1999), about an American GI who travels to Budapest to visit the bath houses that he has heard about from a French fellow soldier and finds that they bring out his passionate side and enable himself to find his real (gay) sexual self; and *8mm 2* (2005), the story of a young couple whose sexual adventures in Budapest, which include a threesome with a local model, lead them to be blackmailed and pitched into a world of violence and terror. Other films have used spa locations to suggest old-fashioned elegance and opulence. The Grandhotel Pupp in Karlovy Vary, which regained its original name in 1989, featured in the 2006 James Bond film *Casino Royale*. Its façade was also used, along with that of the nearby Bristol Palace Hotel, in *The Grand Budapest Hotel* (2014), much of which was actually filmed in abandoned thermal baths in Görlitz in Germany.

While heritage enthusiasts and film-makers have been evoking their past glories and excesses, forward-looking managements have been busily reinventing Europe's leading historic spas as conference and congress centres and equipping them to cater for the new seemingly insatiable global demand for wellness. The first two decades of the twenty-first century have seen traditional spas embrace health and leisure tourism by focusing increasingly on de-stressing and detoxing wellness packages and beauty treatments. This has meant a significant readjustment in terms of guests and staff. The average length of stay for spa guests has plummeted from three to four weeks to three to four days. There are fewer doctors and medical personnel and more fitness and lifestyle coaches, personal trainers, and massage and beauty therapists. Major investment in brand-new facilities is changing the physical appearance as well as the atmosphere of many of the spas that have featured in this book. Ultra-modern thermal complexes using the thermal mineral waters in swimming pools, Jacuzzis and other leisure facilities, but also providing treatment rooms, have replaced nineteenth-century bath houses. Some have been built on the site of earlier spa buildings, like the new Römertherme in Baden bei Wien (1999), the Caracalla

Therme in Baden-Baden, the Thermae Bath Spa (2006), the Salzkammergut Therme in Bad Ischl (2008) and the new Tamina Therme in Bad Ragaz (2009). Others are on brand-new sites, like the Thermes de Spa erected on top of the hill above the town of Spa in 2004 and reached by cable railway, and the Emser Therme built next to the old bath house in Bad Ems in 2012.

There is a certain bland sameness and clinical cleanliness about these ultra-modern thermal establishments. With their open-plan design, bright uniform lighting and piped music, they lack the dark hidden corners and the live entertainment of the old bath houses they have replaced and do not offer the same opportunities for *Kurschatten*. Just occasionally in recent years there have been echoes in historic spas of the more decadent activities of past centuries. The Gellért Hotel in Budapest gained notoriety in 2011 for hosting a sex party for a German insurance company with prostitutes wearing colour-coded wristbands according to which level of executives they were pleasuring. This throwback to the nineteenth century, when accounts refer to 'women of ill fame' frequenting the Gellért Baths and renting out furnished rooms above them to entertain their clients, was exceptional, however. Overwhelmingly over the last hundred years across Europe's spas the balance has swung away from hedonism towards health, or rather wellness.

CONCLUSION – EUROPE'S TRADITIONAL SPAS TODAY

Europe's traditional spas are still doing what they have always done, pandering to a widespread appetite for health, hedonism and hypochondria, presenting themselves as Utopian sanctuaries and playing to rich people's dreams and fantasies of reversing the ageing process and recapturing lost youth. The illnesses which they claim to treat may have changed but the claims about their curative potential have not. There is not much mention nowadays of gout or neurasthenia. Rather the emphasis is on stress and burnout, or what the glossy brochure about the curative powers of the 'yellow gold' of Baden bei Wien's sulphurous waters calls 'chronic civilisation diseases'.

Nowadays they are just a relatively small part of the $4.2 trillion (£3.4 trillion) global wellness industry in which the emphasis has shifted away from the inland spas of Europe to beach resorts in Asia, Africa, the Caribbean and Latin America. A list of the ten best spas for men in *The Times* in 2018 largely featured places in India, Mexico, Morocco and Vietnam. In listings confined to Europe, spas in the Mediterranean south score heavily over the traditional *Kurorte* and *villes d'eaux* of Germany, Austria, Bohemia, Switzerland and France. A 2018 *Times* guide to the best spas in Europe for wellness holidays was dominated by resorts in Greece, Crete, Menorca and Portugal. Not one of the spas featured in this book appeared in either of these lists.

In response to these trends, the historic European spas have incorporated more exotic and specifically Eastern techniques and therapies into their range of treatments. Many now offer Shiatsu massage, various types of yoga and Buddhist-style mindfulness and meditation programmes. The top floor of the former Kaiserflügel in the old *Kurhaus* in Bad Ems, where Wilhelm I stayed for his twenty cures, is now occupied by the Maharishi Ayurveda Health Centre. Based on the principles of the Maharishi Mahesh Yogi, the Indian guru credited with founding transcendental meditation and famous for being visited by the Beatles, it offers 'the golden path to health, youthfulness and joy of life' providing 'prevention, rejuvenation, revitalisation and cure'. The centre offers a series of programmes ranging from a three-day regeneration weekend to a twenty-one-day Panchakarma health vacation. It claims that two weeks of Panchakarma will reduce the risk of a heart attack by 17.8 per cent and eliminate 50 per cent of the toxins in the bloodstream, while practising ayurveda techniques over a period of ten months, including a ten-day Panchakarma treatment at Bad Ems, will lead to a reduction in biological age of 4.8 years. When I stayed in Bad Ems in 2018, forty-four people were taking part in one of these programmes, considerably outnumbering guests taking more traditional spa cures in the adjoining Häcker's Grand Hotel.

In other respects, Europe's historic spas have preserved a more traditional approach. Indeed the modern emphasis on wellness has brought a return to the classical idea of spas as places for cultivating all-round fitness. With their gyms and exercise rooms often attracting as many guests and occupying as much space as their pools, modern spa hotels have reverted to the role of the bath complexes and gymnasia of the ancient Greeks and Romans. The serious medical side is also very much to the fore today. Those who are ill still come for prescribed courses of treatment paid for either out of social insurance or privately. This is especially the case in Eastern European countries where medical tourism is an important foreign-currency earner. It is one of three key 'product lines' promoted by the Czech tourist authority alongside cultural and active tourism. There are still lots of spa buildings and sanatoria full of long corridors where patients sit waiting on plastic chairs clutching their treatment plans and white-coated doctors and therapists pop in and out of small cubicles containing individual baths, massage tables, inhalation chambers and electrical equipment of various kinds. In that respect, it remains a rather hidden world.

There have, of course, been changes over the years. There is a much greater emphasis nowadays on health and safety, hygiene and cleanliness. Gone are the filthy pools full of scum and the remnants of suppurating wounds so graphically described by visitors to spas in previous centuries. The water in some baths is now treated with so much chlorine that the effect of the minerals in them has been largely dissipated. There is some evidence of a fightback against this trend. In 2018, for the first time, the Sandford Parks Lido, an open-air swimming pool in Cheltenham, was filled with the natural thermal water which bubbles up from the ground rather than with heavily chlorinated mains water. But so far this is a rare challenge to the ultra-cautious health and safety culture. Hygiene concerns have stopped drinking of the waters at another British spa. Analysis of Harrogate's water in 2012 revealed it to have two and a half times the permitted level of arsenic. The tap outside the old Royal Pump Room was immediately turned off, prompting protests from local historians and spa enthusiasts who pointed out that the water's composition had been the same for hundreds of years with no apparent ill effects to those who had imbibed it. It has now been turned on again although a notice above the tap indicates that the water should not be drunk. Overall, drinking mineral waters at source, rather than in bottled form, has become less popular, often again because of perceived safety issues. Maybe the rising concern about single-use plastic bottles will lead us back to drinking from fountains again.

Another clear trend is for spa treatments to be softer and less punishing than they used to be. I can testify to this in terms of my own experiences of massages over the last four decades. On my visits to the spas of Hungary and Yugoslavia in the mid-1980s, I usually received a satisfyingly thorough pummelling, often from a lady of Amazonian proportions. I have particularly vivid memories of one such in Yugoslavia clad in a huge rubber apron powerfully directing jets of cold water at me as she fired questions about the British royal family. The male masseurs were built along similarly sturdy lines. I recall lying on a bare steel table resembling a gurney in a subterranean chamber off the Gellért Baths being alternately pummelled and hosed down by a man with a bullet head and enormous belly dripping in sweat and wearing just a loincloth. When I returned there in 2016 the room had been turned into a relaxation area with loungers – the gurney-like tables had disappeared, as had the masseur. Those administering massages, who are now almost invariably called therapists, have become noticeably lighter of both build and touch over the years. I fear it is all part of the modern spa ethos of pampering rather than punishing.

The aristocratic atmosphere that once pervaded Europe's leading spas has also gone. Even where they survive, monarchs and the nobility no longer patronise them and the buildings where once they resided have been turned to other uses. The Englischer Hof, halfway along the Römerstrasse in Bad Ems and once one of the town's grandest hotels whose guests included Leopold and several other crowned heads, is now the Malberg Klinik into which as I passed a woman was being wheeled in from an ambulance. It specialises in rehabilitation treatment for those with cancer, diabetes and conditions of the ear, nose and throat. The ground floor resembles a hospital waiting area with a rather grim canteen serving unappetising-looking meals. How different from its heyday as the chosen lodging place of the English upper-class *Kurgäste*.

Yet at the same time Europe's leading historic spas are still catering for a distinctly upmarket clientele. They are home to some of Europe's grandest and most luxurious hotels: Brenners Park Hotel in Baden-Baden, Hotel Célestins in Vichy, Häcker's Grand Hotel in Bad Ems, Grandhotel Pupp in Karlovy Vary, the Nové Lázně in Mariánské Lázně and the Grand Resort in Bad Ragaz. These hotels are increasingly attracting wealthy Middle Eastern guests, predominantly coming for rehabilitation and medical treatment, and a growing number of Russians, just as they did in the mid-nineteenth century. Sascha Häcker, owner and manager of Häcker's Grand Hotel in Bad Ems, told me that he sees the Russians as the future saviours of the traditional *Kurorte*. Their passion for both health and hedonism would certainly seem to make them the ideal spa guests. In the words of Stephan Wagner, Director of Spa and Wellbeing at the Grand Resort Bad Ragaz, where twenty-four Russian travel agents were being entertained during my stay, 'The Russians know how to party but they also know how to look after their bodies.'

The grand hotels, and the numerous more modest establishments which continue to welcome guests to Europe's traditional spas, offer a combination of medical treatments and wellness and beauty packages. The latter predominate, typically providing three to five days of pampering, tailored to cash-rich but time-short baby boomers and members of Generation X who make up many of their guests. Traditional spa therapies such as baths, douches, massages, mud packs and inhalations are complemented by new ones like cryotherapy which involves freezing the body through one- to three-minute blasts of liquid nitrogen. Those booking in for longer and more serious medical cures are in a minority. Few now come to a spa for the two- or three-month stay that was the norm in the eighteenth and nineteenth centuries. Many do not even manage three weeks, although that is still posited as the minimum period for a real cure to have any effect and it remains the preferred duration for those undergoing rehabilitation and more serious medical treatments in the sanatoria which are still to be found tucked away on the periphery of *Kurparks*.

What Europe's traditional spas can offer which the newer Asian and African resorts cannot is history and heritage. This is rightly being highlighted with initiatives like the granting of UNESCO World Heritage status and through marketing which emphasises their historical interest and architectural treasures. Many spa towns now host major arts festivals and cultural events. To some extent this is reviving their role as the cafés of Europe, attracting writers, artists, composers and other creative figures. Former residences, bath houses, drinking halls and assembly rooms are being turned into artists' colonies, galleries, concert halls and performance spaces. It may be that the future for several Continental spas lies in following the lead taken by British watering places like Bath, Cheltenham, Buxton and Harrogate, and becoming cultural centres rather than continuing as health resorts. For the time being, however, these two roles exist side by side, just as they have for several centuries, with entertainment, diversions and distractions proving as much of a draw for guests as the waters and the cure.

The familiar ambiguities and tensions which have long been at the heart of spa life remain. One such is the juxtaposition of desperation and decadence, represented by the close proximity of the seriously ill in search of a cure and those who have come just to relax and chill out. I was acutely aware of this during a stay in the Sebastianeum in Bad Wörishofen (the prefix Bad, usually only given to places with natural mineral water springs, was granted in 1920 by the Bavarian state in recognition of the town's significant contribution to balneology). There is a very clear divide between the majority of guests, who are well heeled, fit and essentially taking a healthy and relaxing holiday, and the minority who have serious medical conditions and have been sent by their doctors for a cure paid for out of social insurance. Those in the latter group manoeuvre themselves around cautiously on crutches or in wheelchairs, looking weary and dejected. I had a long and moving conversation with one of them, whose sad face had haunted me across the dining room. She was suffering from a serious muscle-wasting disease and clearly in considerable pain. She told me her grim life story: her parents had divorced when she was young, she herself had brought up two children as a single mother, and her illness had been exacerbated by stress and over-prescription of cortisone. She thanked God that she had been sent to Bad Wörishofen for a free cure but it was clear that she felt understandably envious of her fellow Kurgäste who were healthy, affluent and sitting nearby drinking large glasses of beer and wine. 'Because you paid, you will have had a half hour with the doctor,' she said to me. 'I only got ten minutes.'

The contrast between the sickly state of patients and the vigorous health of the staff that so struck Prince Shcherbátsky on his visit to Bad Soden in *Anna Karenina* is also still very evident today. In Bad Ems those walking along the Römerstrasse are divided between dangerously obese or painfully thin figures with pallid skin and downcast expressions shuffling along in ill-fitting tracksuits and old trainers, often puffing on cigarettes, and vigorous, jaunty young men and women in neatly pressed spotless white trousers and brightly coloured jackets advertising the clinic where they work as therapists. Here, too, there continues to be a very clear segregation between the healthy and the sick. The latter are mostly hidden away in three vast sanatoria in a wooded area known as the *Kurwald* at the top of the steep hill above the town, accessed by a cable railway. A notice greeting visitors exiting at the upper station proposes 'a wander round the clinics'. This somewhat bizarre tourist attraction is really only for the most dedicated devotees of spa medicine. It involves a walk past three enormous and very ugly clinics, one named after Paracelsus, each with over 200 beds. They are filled with patients paid for by social insurance schemes, who are either recovering from operations or taking cures to help ease conditions ranging from cancer to depression. Tourists brave enough to enter the reception areas of these vast buildings are greeted with a pervasive odour of boiled cabbage emanating from their ground-floor cafeterias.

Concern that the presence of those who are sick does not disturb other more able-bodied guests continues to be a major preoccupation of those who run spa establishments. Indeed, it has become even more important when so many spas are in the business of promoting and packaging wellness. As the Director of Wellbeing at one of the leading spa hotels candidly put it as he led me round its medical facilities: 'We don't want very ill people here. It's all right to see people going round on crutches but guests coming on a wellness package do not want to see very ill people around them.'

Another familiar theme, the close proximity of health and hedonism, continues to be very evident. It is graphically illustrated in Bad Ems by two rather striking juxtapositions along the Römerstrasse, the main street which runs along the bank of the Lahn. Directly opposite the entrance to the theatre is a shop selling orthopaedic aids with a window display featuring wheelchairs, Zimmer frames, commodes, walking sticks and orthopaedic shoes. A few yards along the street, directly opposite the entrance to the casino, which is unusually for nowadays an entirely smoking area, another medical supplier displays oxygen masks and breathing apparatus. There might as well be a sign warning those about to light up and place their bets of the wages of sin. In fact, the casino in Spa does make a very clear attempt to warn would-be clients of the dangers that lurk around its tables. Prominently displayed in the entrance lobby is a booklet about the serious risks and effects of addiction to gambling. It includes a form that you can fill in to get banned from all casinos in Belgium and so save yourself from this potentially dangerous affliction.

Overall, the casinos which were once one of the chief draws for visitors to European spas are now in a sorry state. Together with official unease about their role in fuelling addiction, the huge rise in online gambling has largely killed off their appeal. Their extravagant and opulent décor has been ruined by the installation of rows of garish fruit machines and huge electronic screens flashing up details of prizes and promotions. In Baden-Baden and Baden bei Wien the casinos, largely frequented by Russian and Chinese patrons, still have a faint whiff of glamour and sophistication and manage to preserve some kind of formal dress code. Yet even here more people are to be found in the restaurant and bar areas than around the gaming tables. Other traditional spa casinos have given up on a dress code and are now a pale shadow of what they once were, their grand halls largely empty with often just a handful of figures in scruffy anoraks hunched over slot machines. In an effort to encourage custom the casino at Spa provides a self-service cafeteria offering free soup, crisps, tea, coffee and soft drinks. During my Saturday evening visit, I was the only person to avail myself of these facilities. The whole place was largely deserted with just a few determined and impassive men playing roulette and poker in an upstairs room. The casino at Bad Ems, which only reopened in 1987 in a rather unattractive extension to the *Kursaal*, was even emptier when I called in one weekday evening. Less than half a dozen punters were feeding coins into the ubiquitous slot machines which now occupy most of the floor space. The room devoted to roulette and blackjack, the only card game on offer, did not attract a single visitor during the two hours I spent there. Occasionally an exceptionally bored-looking croupier would spin the roulette wheel to conform with legal requirements but otherwise absolutely nothing was going on. The bar attendant told me I was his only customer of the evening – I went wild and had one small mineral water – and said that the staff looked back fondly to pre-internet days when the place was buzzing with life. The casino is currently open every day from 1 p.m. to 2.30 a.m. for 'automatic games' and from 7 p.m. to 2.30 a.m. for 'classic games' but he wondered how long the latter will survive and, indeed, if the casino as a whole has much of a future. Sascha Häcker, whose hotel is just a few hundred yards away, would like to see the casino reinvent itself and try to rekindle some of its former glamour with dance shows, ladies' nights and formal champagne receptions. I think it will take more than that to attract the kind of clientele and the numbers described as crowding spa casinos in mid-nineteenth-century novels. It will be especially difficult, I suspect, to win back female gamblers of the kind who feature so prominently in *Can You Forgive Her?*, *Daniel Deronda* and 'Eugene Pickering'.

If gambling is in steep decline, then so too is flirting. There is little evidence of clandestine romances and affairs among the largely middle-aged or elderly *curistes* and *Kurgäste* who frequent the spas of Europe today. There is a significant preponderance of single women aged between sixty-five and ninety. They have usually been my companions at meals where our conversations have largely revolved around our various ailments and treatments and the quality of the food. The only frisson, if such it can be called, has come when there has been a mild dispute as to the ownership of the various identical bottles of mineral water which are kept on a shelf by the table to be reclaimed at each meal. This can be avoided by the simple expedient of initialling or otherwise marking the label of one's own bottle. Neither in the dining rooms, nor in the baths or drinking halls of the spas that I have visited over recent years, have I been aware of any romantic undercurrents. The diversions and entertainments which formerly lent themselves to *Kurschatten* fantasies and experiences, strolls around the *Kurparks*, morning and afternoon *Kurkonzerte* and visits to cafés to mitigate the severity of the cure regime with a little coffee, cake and ice cream, are still prominent features of spa life but they do not seem to stimulate the amatory impulses that they once did.

There is one respect in which spas have become slightly more daring in recent years. Several have reverted to mixed bathing after a long period of segregating the sexes. The Gellért Baths threw open their formerly separate male and female thermal pools to both sexes in 2013. It does not seem to have produced an outburst of immorality. A complex and comprehensive set of by-laws displayed in the magnificent glass-roofed entrance hall prohibit any kind of sexual activity or soliciting. The other Budapest baths offer sessions of either mixed or single-sex bathing on different days. Most Continental spas have clung defiantly to dispensing with swimming costumes for steam rooms, saunas and small plunge pools, a practice that often catches out and sometimes unsettles British and American visitors. The first floor of the Thermes de Spa offers a choice of either nude or covered bathing. I was roundly rebuked when entering the steam room of the nude side with my swimming trunks on, having failed to grasp the full import of the word '*naturel*' at the door, and had hastily to remove them. There is no sign of this enforced nudity encouraging any of the 'wanton dalliances' which so scandalised visitors to spas in centuries gone by.

With both gambling and flirting so curtailed, the most hedonistic aspect of spas nowadays is to be found in the nature of some of the treatments on offer. In the Gellért Baths you can bathe in a private thermal water pool into which a bottle of red wine has been poured or take a Cleopatra Bath, where milk and honey are added to the water. The Thermal Spa Menu at the Grand Resort Bad Ragaz includes facial treatments using white caviar. Other spas offer similarly self-indulgent treatments, while marginally less decadent delights are to be found in the relaxation rooms where you end up at the end of your progress through baths, saunas, steam rooms and plunge pools. The Friedrichsbad in Baden-Baden has an amazing Blue Room with blue fibreglass beds which follow the contours of the human body. From loudspeakers around the head area emanate strange electronic echoes and vibrations, possibly based on dolphin cries which are a favourite sound effect in such places. The blue ceiling enhances the feeling that you are under water. The Thermes de Spa has a chilling-out room on the non-nude side where the lighting picks out and enhances white and light colours. Bikinis particularly are made to glow in the dark with an exciting and dazzling effect of which Casanova would undoubtedly have approved.

With health still very much to the fore, albeit increasingly in the guise of wellness, and hedonism not completely banished, what of that third essential element in spa culture, hypochondria? It has not disappeared even if it is not quite what it was. Spas remain the perfect places for hypochondriacs to indulge their imagined illnesses and neuroses. They are full of doctors, especially psychotherapists and analysts of various kinds specialising in treating stress, burnout and psychosomatic illnesses. They have the time to listen to their patients and will not tell them brusquely to go away and pull themselves together. There will always be plenty of fellow sufferers with whom to discuss your symptoms and phobias. To that extent, spas do remain a paradise for hypochondriacs and valetudinarians.

Perhaps the best way to end this hidden history of spas is with a brief report on the current state of some of the main ones that have featured in this book, based on my own recent stays in them.

In Bath a fourth 'h' in the form of heritage has taken the place of health, hedonism and hypochondria. The city was declared a UNESCO World Heritage site in 1987 and has effectively turned itself into a highly successful tourist trap, attracting over 330,000 international visitors spending around £420 million annually. Among the leading visitor attractions are the superbly presented Roman Baths complex and the Jane Austen Experience where you can dress up in Regency costume, try your hand at writing with quill and ink, play parlour games of the kind that might have amused the Company in the eighteenth century and, of course, take elegant afternoon tea. Although there are no longer any serious medical treatments on offer, it is possible once again to taste the thermal mineral water from fountains in the Pump Room and the adjoining West baths and to swim in it in the Bath Thermae Spa with its atmospheric rooftop pool offering views over the Georgian city. The experience is altogether cleaner and more comfortable than that described by those taking a cure in its eighteenth- and early nineteenth-century heyday.

Spa, which similarly no longer provides cures or treatments, is also seeking to promote itself primarily as a historical heritage site. The old nineteenth-century baths lie derelict and forlorn in the middle of the town, the action having moved to the ultra-modern hilltop Thermes de Spa. The once elegant Parc des Sept Heures, laid out in 1758 and so called because that was the time when *curistes* would promenade there, is now distinctly scruffy and the Galerie Leopold II at its centre has become a haunt for winos and disaffected teenagers. The house where Queen Marie Henriette of Belgium spent her latter years after finally escaping from her philandering husband, still known as the Villa Royale, has been turned into a museum charting the town's history as a spa and the former Proudhon Pump Room houses the tourist office as well as a drinking fountain. You can still take the waters at the sources dotted around the outskirts of the town – most have an adjoining restaurant occupying the old pump room – but they are virtually deserted. On the morning I spent going round them, I did not meet a single other person. Bottling water remains one of the main local industries. You can visit the gallery of the Spa Monopole factory and watch 66,000 bottles an hour being filled on automated conveyor belts below. Three strengths are produced: *Reine*, a still water which comes from the Marie Henriette spring; *Finesse*, a light sparkling variety; and *Intense*, a more highly carbonated water. The exhibition in the bottling plant behind the town railway station is full of interesting facts about water. It must be one of the few tourist attractions in the world to make a virtue of locally high levels of rainfall, proudly pointing out that the Spa region receives one and a half times more rain than the Belgian average.

Baden bei Wien retains much of its charm with a traffic-free central area and a delightful *Kurpark*, at the entrance to which are three traditional British-style telephone boxes and an old-fashioned weighing machine. Operetta still flourishes here with performances in the Sommerarena with its retractable roof and in the Stadttheater, and in the summer you can sit under the chestnut trees in the *Kurpark* listening to the *Kurorchester* playing waltzes, polkas and marches by the composers who lived in the town during its belle époque. There are still several sanatoria operated by trade unions providing cures for their members but cuts in social security budgets have reduced the annual number of *Kurgäste* from a peak of 600,000 to around 450,000 and several hotels in the town have recently closed. Spa treatments are carried out in a large clinical complex, the Badener Kurzentrum, adjoining the modern Römertherme, which is designed for leisure swimming, and you can also bathe in the naturally hot sulphurous waters in the open-air Thermal Strandbad. The old bath houses dotted around the town, which were mostly closed in the 1970s, have found alternative uses: the Leopoldsbad as the tourist information centre, the Franzensbad as a Turkish bath, the Josefbad as a café, the Marienquelle as a clinic, while the Sauerhofbad and Herzogbad have been incorporated into hotels. The elegant neoclassical Frauenbad, dating from 1821, houses a museum dedicated to the work of the locally born artist, Arnulf Rainer. His brutalist, angst-ridden paintings, which often involve daubing black or red splodges over photographs based on images of nineteenth-century mental patients, contrast with the cool grey marble of the old bath house but perhaps speak powerfully in their own way of the hidden shadow side of spa life.

The spa district of Baden bei Zürich is currently undergoing total renovation. The baths and three adjoining spa hotels, including the Verenahof where Hermann Hesse stayed annually for more than twenty-five years, were closed some years ago and are scheduled to reopen in 2021 as an ultra-modern thermal baths complex, seventy-room rehabilitation clinic and medical centre, together with thirty-eight apartments. Meanwhile you can still sit on the red bench set against the back wall of the former Inhalatorium, which now houses physiotherapy and medical practices, and dangle your feet in the thermal water while looking out on the fast-flowing waters of the River Limmat. There is also a small temporary outdoor bath for public use in the *Kurplatz* in front of the Hotel Blume. If you stay in that hotel, which dates from 1421 and has an atmospheric central atrium with one of the oldest working lifts in Switzerland, you can wallow in thermal water in one of the old baths set into the floor in the basement. Staff will run you one at twenty minutes' notice. The walk from the town station to the spa and hotel quarter affords a striking illustration of the continuing juxtaposition of health and hedonism. On the right side of the Bäderstrasse stands a rather forbidding grey building which was once a spa hotel and now houses a rehabilitation clinic. Opposite is the casino, where 'over 320 different state-of-the-art slot machines provide an electrifying atmosphere' along with the more traditional attractions of roulette, poker, blackjack and two games devised in Baden, Big Shot, played with dice, and Black James, a variation on blackjack.

Bad Ragaz continues to make good use of the thermal water from the Tamina Gorge. It is pumped directly to the Dorfbad in the centre of the small town and to the Grand Resort Bad Ragaz, set in a *Kurpark* on its outskirts and incorporating the Quellenhof and Hof hotels. The Dorfbad, built in 1866 with an elegant colonnaded neoclassical façade, now houses the Tourist Information Centre and the Spahouse Bad Ragaz and Schaub Institute, an alternative medicine centre offering a variety of natural therapies and wellness treatments. Its old individual bath rooms have been imaginatively decorated and individually themed – there is a philosopher's bath, the walls of which are covered with suitably profound quotations – and are popular for romantic evening candle-lit meals as well as hydrotherapy sessions. While showing me round, the director, Stefan Schaub, took particular delight in extracting from a cupboard a jar in which five large leeches were squirming around. He regularly uses them in treating varicose veins, thrombosis and other conditions where he says their bloodletting properties are invaluable. It is good, if slightly off-putting, to see a traditional spa remedy still being applied.

There is no mention of leeches in the extensive spa treatment menu at the Grand Resort Bad Ragaz, which presents itself as 'Europe's Leading Wellbeing & Medical Health Resort' and offers high-end health and hedonism, with the accent firmly on the former. Thermal water supplies the elegant Helena Bath, built in 1923, a large sports pool used for aqua exercise classes and serious swimming, a children's pool in the family spa area and an outdoor garden pool as well as the extensive indoor and outdoor baths of varying temperatures in the adjoining public Tamina Therme. Alongside its two five-star hotels, six gourmet restaurants and shopping mall with jewellery and clothes boutiques, the Resort also houses a medical centre offering consultations and treatments in a wide variety of specialities, including orthopaedics, rheumatology, gynaecology, dermatology, internal medicine and cardiology. It is, indeed, a spa town in miniature.

At the centre of the Resort is the nine-storey Spa Tower, built in 2008. Its lower floors house a twenty-five-bed clinic with twenty-four-hour nursing care largely used by patients recovering from operations and cancer treatment. The upper floors are given over to spacious spa suites, fitted out with huge Jacuzzi-style baths fed directly from the Tamina spring. Guests staying here will find that the minibars are stocked entirely with bottled waters and soft drinks (they may also find, as I did, a Russian *Men Only*-style magazine left by a previous occupant on the top shelf of the huge wardrobe – a rare throwback to old-style spa *Kurschatten* in what is otherwise an unimpeachably pure, clinical and spotless environment). Indeed, there is not a drop of alcohol to be had in the building. The bar on the ground floor is presided over by Irina Taculina, the water sommelière, who offers tastings of twenty bottled waters, ranging from one sourced from a Norwegian glacier, which tastes remarkably like London tap water, to others with a high mineral content from the mountains of Switzerland, Wales and Catalonia. As she cheerfully cracks open the bottles, she dispenses useful advice: drink sparkling water as an aperitif before a meal because it opens the taste buds, but still water while eating; use water with a low mineral content for detoxing, but one with plenty of minerals in it for cooking.

This watery theme extends across the Resort. The blue carpets in the bedrooms and corridors are designed to represent flowing streams and waves and the decorations in the public rooms are modelled on rain droplets and waterfalls. A carafe of Tamina thermal water is served with every meal and the Asian restaurant is called Namun, the Thai word for hot water. In the words of Anita Basu, director of the medical centre, which has its own thermal mineral water pool for hydrotherapy and balneology, 'water is our DNA.' This theme is taken up with some alacrity by one of her staff, Dr Matthias Fenzl, who specialises in sports medicine, when I meet him over a glass of water in the hotel bar. He comes armed with references to academic papers pointing to the benefits of immersion and exercise in water for the cardiovascular and musculoskeletal systems and regularly leaps up from his seat to demonstrate, walking fast forwards and backwards while slowly circling his arms – precisely the movements that I had been undertaking in the early-morning Aquafit class in the sports pool. When we part, he presents me with a copy of his book, *Aqua-Training Schlägt Wellen*, which is packed with pictures of lithe figures flexing their muscles under water. His enthusiasm reminds me of Dr Seremet in Kiseljak thirty-five years ago (see page 243). It is good to know that there are still such dedicated 'water doctors' around in the spas of Europe.

Not surprisingly, water features prominently in the Resort's two most popular wellness packages, devoted to detoxing and weight loss. The daily regime for those taking them, as outlined to me by Stephan Wagner, Director of Spa and Wellbeing, begins with an early-morning drink of warm water, an 8 a.m. session of aquagym and a light breakfast, followed later in the day by a twenty-minute soak in the thermal pool, various treatments including Kneipp-style wrappings, a carefully controlled diet and the consumption of at least two litres of Ragazer thermal water. There are also intravenous vitamin infusions and a procedure known as chelation which binds together and expels heavy metals. Wagner practises what he preaches. When I met him for lunch in the Verve restaurant, whose motto is 'healthy cuisine without sacrifice', he was himself in the middle of a four-day detox. For both of us it was a liquid lunch consisting of a small bowl of consommé and a glass of mineral water. He insisted that his was still and served at room temperature. I am afraid that I ignored sommelière Irina's advice and splashed out on a small bottle of a slightly chilled sparkling variety from the Jura mountains.

Of the three spa treatments I was able to squeeze into an all-too-brief stay here, only one used water. This was the Haki Flow Deluxe, which was carried out in the main pool of the Tamina Therme at

6.45 in the morning before it opened for the day. Devised by an Austrian therapist, Harald Kitz, it involved lying on my back floating in the thermal water while being cradled and gently manipulated by the manager of the Therme's wellness department. He told me that it was particularly good for those who think too much and have 'lots of stuff in their heads' – in which case I was a prime candidate to benefit from it – but I have to confess that while it was relaxing I was rather preoccupied by the pressure of water in my ears, which were permanently submerged. Despite its name, my Tamina flow massage had no watery element but was thorough and satisfying, more like physiotherapy in that it included some manipulation and rotation of the arms and legs. My third treatment, a Chi Nei Tsang massage, was the most challenging. Part of the detox programme, it involves considerable pressure being applied in turn to the organs in the abdomen. The aim is temporarily to block the blood supply to them, so that when it is restored it is with an increased force which supposedly releases and expels toxins. The diminutive therapist warned me that it would be painful, as indeed it was, but I steeled myself with the maxim of 'no pain, no gain' which has inspired so many spa patients over the centuries. Alas, I had no real chance to measure its effects as I proceeded almost immediately afterwards to enjoy a huge Thai meal of shrimp dim sum, crispy duck, egg noodles and spicy vegetables in the Namun restaurant washed down with copious quantities of thermal water. In providing opportunities for such dramatic swings from self-punishment to self-indulgence, as part of its commitment to combining serious health and wellness regimes with unashamed luxury, the Grand Resort at Bad Ragaz still wonderfully evokes the essence and the ambiguity of the spa experience as it has played out in the traditional European *Kurorte* over the last three centuries. More specifically, it offers a taste of both the elegance and the over-the-top extravagance of spas in their belle époque.

Bad Ischl offers more modest if equally nostalgic pleasures. It continues to capitalise on its long connection with Franz Joseph who remains a ubiquitous presence around the town. There is a life-size depiction of him as a young man in military uniform perched somewhat incongruously above a photographic shop in the Kreuzplatz and another statue, in which he appears in full hunting gear with a dead deer at his feet, just off a path beside the River Traun. When I last visited, there was also a rather splendid cut-out figure of the emperor pushing a mowing machine in the riverside gardens, with his wife Sisi tending the nearby flowerbed. His birthday on 18 August is celebrated every year with a lavish *Kaiserfest*, which involves an actor dressed as Franz Joseph arriving by steam train and parading through the town, and a Mass in the parish church at which, exceptionally, the old Austrian imperial hymn (*'Gott erhalte Franz den Kaiser'*, *God save Franz, the emperor*) is allowed to be sung. The Habsburg family still live in a wing of the Kaiservilla, which is open to the public. The guides will tell you all about Sisi's exercise regime to preserve her wasp waist and Franz Joseph's spartan lifestyle, which involved a jug of hot water being brought to him at 3.30 every morning for his ablutions, but, as I discovered, they clam up when asked about the whereabouts of the secret doorway that led to Katharina Schratt's adjoining villa. Like Baden bei Wien, Bad Ischl has an annual operetta festival, held in the Lehár Theatre in the middle of the *Kurpark*. A quartet of Slovakian musicians plays every day either in the *Kurpark* or in Zauner's café on the esplanade overlooking the Traun, where I have whiled away many a pleasant hour sipping iced coffee and guzzling chocolate and apricot cake while looking across to Franz Lehár's villa on the other side of the river. It is possible to bathe in the saline waters and undertake medical and wellness treatments in the modern Salzkammergut-Therme and adjoining EurothermenResort, which boasts a brine grotto and advertises its sauna suite with the strapline 'Sweat like an Emperor'. But essentially this is a spa town which focuses on heritage more than on health, and is all the more appealing for so doing.

Baden-Baden remains one of the most opulent and elegant of Europe's spa resorts. The magnificent arcaded mid-nineteenth-century

Trinkhalle in the Kaiserallee now serves as the tourist office and also provides fountains for sampling the thermal waters. Its casino, described by Marlene Dietrich as the most beautiful in the world, is not in quite such a sorry state as those in other spas and retains something of the chic and glamour of its glory days, although even here, when I last visited more people were watching the Netherlands playing Russia in the European Cup on television screens than were gathered round the roulette wheels or card tables. Walking down the Lichtentaler Allee past the busts of Turgenev, Clara Schumann and Brahms, and the sixty-four different varieties of dahlias in the flower beds, you meet immaculately coiffed and made-up elderly ladies, with immaculately groomed little dogs trotting along beside them. In the Friedrichsbad Baden-Baden still offers perhaps the most authentic and invigorating spa bathing experience anywhere in Europe. Men and women proceed separately through the first twelve stages of the complex bathing ritual, which includes a vigorous scrub down with a brush and olive soap as well as immersion in pools and steam rooms of varying temperatures, before joining for a grand unisex finale in a circular pool under the huge central dome.

The two towns associated with the birth and development of hydrotherapy have more of a feel of being working spas. The former Graefenberg, now called Jeseník and situated on the Czech–Polish border, still has a number of sanatoria specialising in the treatments which Vincent Priessnitz pioneered there, including a large and somewhat forbidding one bearing his name. A balneopark opened in 2010 on the hillside behind it encompassing seven water features, including foot baths, jets and showers. The most popular is the 'Priessnitz natural bath for upper and lower limbs' which attracts a steady stream of bathers who strip off their trousers or hitch up their skirts to wade through the ice-cold water. The recommended minimum time in the water is five seconds and the maximum five minutes. I managed twenty seconds before the cold overcame me but most of my Czech companions showed more stamina and remained in the bath for over a minute, making a series of purposeful circuits round the central handrail. Their grim determination gave way to a cheerful communal sense of satisfaction as they sat round the pool drying off their legs in the sun and doubtless reflecting on Priessnitz's maxim that 'the curative effect is not the cold itself but the heat that is subsequently evoked.' A walking trail established in 2005 takes in many of the most interesting fountains and monuments erected by his grateful patients in the wooded hills above the Priessnitz Sanatorium. There is also an interesting museum in the house where he first began his medical practice.

Bad Wörishofen remains a thriving spa resort with 127 hotels and guest houses, several run by religious orders and more than half of which offer full Kneipp cures. The number of *Kurgäste*, which currently stands at over 150,000 a year, is actually increasing although they are staying for a shorter time than they used to, with few able to afford the time or the money to take the full three-week cure still reckoned as most efficacious and most opting to stay for a week or ten days. In 2018 two of the cure centres established by Kneipp, the massive Kneippianum and an adjoining establishment for children to come and stay with their parents, were closed because of the substantial losses they were incurring as a result of the decline in the number of patients being paid for out of social medical insurance. By contrast, the Sebastianeum, which he originally built as a cure home for fellow priests, and is now run by the Barmherzigen Brüder, a German religious order, thrives as a combination of four-star hotel, sanatorium and religious retreat centre and is the place to go to savour the full hydrotherapy experience. Guests are greeted just inside the front door by a large aluminium watering can from which a steady stream of water pours into a tub below. *Güsse*, (cold showers) which are still at the heart of the Kneipp cure, are performed twice a day by efficient and friendly *Bademeisterin* according to a prescription written out by the doctor with whom you have a consultation at the beginning of your stay. Also prescribed is an individually tailored herbal tea mixture delivered to your bedroom in a brown paper bag by a nurse – mine was a rather bitter combination of nettle and willow – of which you are supposed to take a cup four times a day. Another key element of the Kneipp cure is being woken up at 5 a.m. to have wet towels wrapped round your legs or be given an all-over wipe-down with a damp cloth.

Perhaps the distinctive atmosphere of Europe's traditional spas can best be experienced today in those two former Bohemian *Kurorte* which flourished in La Belle Époque. Karlovy Vary and Mariánské Lázně, as Karlsbad and Marienbad are now known, are still very much working spas, offering treatments and cures for urological, gynaecological, respiratory, dermatological and neurological complaints, as well as for arthritis, rheumatism and diabetes. They are increasingly resorted to for rehabilitation following hip and knee replacement operations and, like other spas today, they provide a wide variety of wellness packages and treatments designed to combat stress and the psychological ills associated with modern lifestyles.

Karlovy Vary has shaken off most of its communist associations. The modern drinking hall where people gather to drink from the powerful Vřídlo spring is no longer named after Yuri Gagarin but rather called the Vřídelní Kolonáda. The Hotel Moskva has become the Grandhotel Pupp again and Bath House No. 5 is more commonly referred to as Alžbětiny Lázně, or the Elizabeth Baths. In other respects, the place feels rather charmingly stuck in the mid-1990s. There are still a large number of working telephone boxes dotted around the streets. The museum of waxworks, which occupies the old Anglican church of St Luke's built in 1877 for the large number of English visitors, with memorials on the wall to those who perished while taking the waters, has a decidedly dated atmosphere. John Major is the most recent British prime minister depicted and Ronald Reagan the last American president. Grouped in the apse is the entire British royal family as it was c.1996 complete with Princess Diana and Sarah Ferguson.

Just up the road from St Luke's a large bust of Karl Marx gazes benignly over the fashionable west end of the town and across to the Russian Orthodox church and the Russian consulate. Russians are now flocking back to Karlovy Vary and account for around 60 per cent of foreign visitors, with Germans making up around 30 per cent and Chinese showing increasing interest. Most still come here primarily to take a cure, receiving treatments either at one of the large number of sanatoria-type hotels, or in one of the three surviving bath houses which offer a mixture of self-indulgent pampering and serious medical interventions. Side by side in the list of treatments on offer at the Elizabeth Baths are a purificatory enema, or colonclysma, and a romantic Sissi (sic) Bath. The former involves Karlovy Vary water being applied 'per rectum to purge the colon', a procedure which is described as 'beneficial in cases of dysfunctions in defecation (constipation) and intestinal disorders (bloating, irregular bowel movements and intestinal dyspepsia)'. The Sissi Bath, by contrast, is simply presented as 'a pearl bath in hot mineral water for two persons surrounded by romantic atmosphere with candles'. Also on offer are irrigation of the gums, intestines and vagina. The gum procedure utilises a special mouthpiece in the shape of a horseshoe perforated with holes through which mineral water is squirted under pressure. Intestinal irrigation involves four to six litres of water being pumped via the colon to remove all solid waste matter sticking to the walls of the intestine, while vaginal irrigation speaks for itself. There is also the pleasingly alliterative if somewhat off-putting-sounding 'paraffin for prostate'. Alongside these serious medical procedures are numerous cosmetic beauty treatments, including champagne face masks, cinnamon wraps, and baths and massages with chocolate, champagne, honey or ginger.

Drinking the waters from one of the twelve springs which have been tapped and are freely available from fountains in elegant pavilions and colonnades remains a popular activity, perhaps more so than in any other spa today. Karlovy Vary's thermal water is promoted for its efficacy in dissolving 'toxic substances which are better excreted in stool, urine, sweat and breath'. A set of guidelines, posted at various points in the town and also in the Spa

Guide Book, lays down that it should be taken only 'after consulting a medical physician with appropriate erudition', drunk just from the traditionally shaped porcelain cups, digested 'while walking slowly', and under no circumstances be used to water plants around the colonnades or discharged on the floor. It also states that 'the drinking cure should be taken when you are relaxed and not in a hurry. It is a small ceremony, during which other people must not be disturbed.' On the whole, these rules are observed. Taking the waters does have the air of a ritual, carried out predominantly in the early morning and early evening with restraint and even reverence. Most people use the distinctive cups, which are sold in little kiosks around the colonnades from around £4, and drink through the long spout in the handle, although there are some who lower the tone by filling up plastic bottles. The girls who once served the water, often wearing mackintoshes to protect themselves from the spray, are long since gone and now everyone has to bend down and serve themselves from one of the fountains which continually gush forth. Prospective drinkers form orderly queues and there is no jostling and little conversation. Having filled their cups, they either promenade through the colonnades or along the streets sipping the water or else sit down in one of the little pavilions. The atmosphere is hushed and serious, very different from what paintings suggest it was like in La Belle Époque when there was considerable conviviality around the springs. I fear that I disobeyed the guidelines by swigging the effervescent warm water, which tastes rather like Alka-Seltzer, somewhat indiscriminately, mixing my drinks by going from spring to spring, and so inducing a bout of diarrhoea.

Karlovy Vary has quite an edgy feel and a surprisingly youthful clientele but its diversions and entertainments are generally respectable and restrained. Several cafés offer dancing – I popped my head into one in the former Military Bath House and saw four middle-aged couples dancing to Abba's 'Mamma Mia' crooned by a young man standing at a keyboard. In common with most spas, it has a disproportionate number of ladies' hat shops and even one selling wigs in a prominent position opposite the Tržní Colonnade. There seems to be a conscious desire to play down its racy past. Alluding to the best-known guest who stayed at what is now Jessenius Hotel along the main Stará Louka Street, the guidebook refers to 'the famous globetrotter Giacomo Casanova', making no mention of the exploits for which he is principally remembered. Goethe and Schiller are similarly recalled in chaste monuments along the path which leads along the riverside from the Grandhotel Pupp to the art gallery and Beethoven stands craggy and hunched in front of the Hotel Richmond, with not a hint of any of their *Kurschatten*.

There is one distinctly decadent and hedonistic pleasure to be had in modern Karlovy Vary. I suspect it is largely aimed at and patronised by the British stag and hen parties which the Czech Republic is attracting in increasing numbers and does not find so many takers among those undertaking a cure or wellness package. Three beer spas have opened in the town over recent years where you can bathe either solo or in a group in a tub full of beer (or in one case in the mash of yeast, hops and malt used for brewing), meanwhile consuming as much light or dark beer as you can imbibe from a tap conveniently positioned next to the tub. The sixty-minute experience, which costs around €70 (£60), ends with a rest on a bed of straw while eating homemade beer bread. It is hard to think of anything less healthy, although the websites of these spas claim that the benefits of bathing in beer include skin rejuvenation, stress reduction, better blood circulation and better heart activity. I have so far resisted the temptation to try it.

Mariánské Lázně, which once had a rather racier reputation, is now very much the staid and sedate country cousin to its more edgy and urban near neighbour. It has an air of geriatric gentility, catering for its largely Russian and German clientele with a range of wellness and rehabilitation packages, plentiful cafés in which to indulge in coffee and cakes, gentle walks through its perfectly maintained parks, and concerts offering light classical and big band music. The main excitement is the eruption every two hours of the Singing

Fountain with its jets of water carefully synchronised to accompany recordings of Céline Dion singing 'My Heart Will Go On' from *Titanic*, the 'Chorus of the Hebrew Slaves' from *Nabucco* and Andrea Bocelli belting out '*Vivo per lei*'. Even more than Karlovy Vary, it gives the impression of being stuck in a time warp. Trolleybuses, of a kind which largely disappeared from Britain's streets in the 1960s, ply the streets. The video shown to visitors to the town museum was made in 1987 and ends with young communist pioneers doing baton-twirling routines. A concert by the local accordion orchestra which I attended in the town's charming theatre featured an eclectic mix of pieces ranging from the 'Radetzky March' to Queen's 'Bohemian Rhapsody', via Édith Piaf and Frank Sinatra. Nothing on the programme was written in the last forty years.

Massive spa hotels lining the main street and dotted around the *Kurpark* are full of elderly Russians and Germans. The one in which I stayed felt like a post-communist care home. Meals are taken communally on shared tables in almost total silence, with even couples exchanging barely a single word, and a stare or at best a wan smile being all that one can expect to receive over the watery soup and sauerkraut. Maybe the lack of conversation has something to do with embarrassment over the fact that the figures one sees across the dinner table have previously been encountered semi-naked or in their dressing gowns queuing up for or receiving treatments in the cavernous corridors of the hotel basement. This is where we all met every morning, clutching our treatment tickets and having filled in a lengthy form declaring that we did not suffer from seventeen different conditions including 'recurrent bleeding of any kind', 'mental status with antisocial symptoms', 'inability to self-care', incontinence or an allergy to cinnamon.

My three treatments all left something to be desired. The first, billed as a 'classic massage', was administered by a sullen masseuse with absolutely no small talk, indeed no talk at all. She simply gestured at me to lie face down on her table and then proceeded to give me the shortest and sloppiest massage that I have ever had. I was smothered with oil (supposedly ginger but it had no discernible smell) which she rubbed over my back and neck using only one hand while 'Some Enchanted Evening' and 'As Time Goes By' played on repeat through loudspeakers on the wall. Very little pressure was applied, my legs, arms, chest and stomach were left untouched, and the whole thing was over in ten minutes, even though my ticket suggested that it should have lasted half an hour.

My next treatment was billed as a 'pearl bath with ginger'. Entering the cubicle for it, I did at least get two words out of the attendant: she pointed reprovingly to my swimming trunks and barked '*Alles aus*' (everything off) before I climbed into a large bath tub full of bubbling water. Once again, the promised ginger seemed conspicuous by its absence. I was left alone to sit in the bath for about twenty-five minutes. With no other distractions, my eye was drawn to the emergency bell pull hovering above me. I was tempted to pull it, if only to enquire about the elusive ginger, but deemed discretion the better part of valour. I had already fallen foul of the attendant in the tiny hotel pool, which was too small to swim in and essentially designed for doing exercises. She rebuked me for putting my flip-flops in the wrong place and bringing into her demesne a blue towel that I had picked up at the entrance instead of an orange one that I should have obtained from her. The heavily regulated regime of the communist era seemed to have lingered here long after the fall of the Iron Curtain.

My third treatment, the most dramatic and scary, was a dry carbon dioxide bath, a modern version of the procedure which so impressed Augustus Granville nearly 200 years ago and which utilises the substantial amounts of CO_2 gas emerging naturally with the water from the swampy ground. After being ushered into a cubicle and taking off my clothes, I climbed into a thick blue plastic bag and lay down on a couch. An attendant appeared, tightened a belt around my chest and then inflated the bag by pumping in CO_2 with a high-pressure hose until I looked and felt like the Michelin Man. She then departed with a cursory '*Gute Nacht*', presumably to induce thoughts of slumber even though it was only ten in the morning. For the next half hour I lay rather uncomfortably in the increasingly sweaty plastic bag. The only sensation I felt was a warmth and tingling in the groin area – something that I suspect Edward VII must have often experienced at Marienbad without needing to go anywhere near a gas bath. I later discovered that, in the words of the medical guide, as well as slowing down the heart rate and lowering blood pressure, 'the gas is also known to stimulate the production of the sexual hormones, which is why it is successful for the improvement of sexual functions and to relieve the menopausal symptoms in women.' At the end of the treatment the attendant returned, greeted me with a brisk '*Guten Morgen*' and asked me to hold my nose as she loosened the belt and the gas escaped. Many of my fellow guests were subjecting themselves to this treatment every morning – once was enough for me.

Drinking the waters remains an important part of the Mariánské Lázně cure although there are fewer people visibly engaged in this activity than in Karlovy Vary. Several of the big spa hotels have their own piped supplies direct from the springs, but the waters are mainly drunk in the elegant neoclassical Pavilion of the Cross Spring which adjoins the magnificent cast-iron Colonnade. Both buildings were substantially reconstructed in the 1980s, when a new pavilion was also built to house the nearby Caroline Spring. As in Karlovy Vary, precise rules govern this aspect of the cure. A small quantity of water from the particular spring prescribed by the doctor should be drunk three times a day before meals, with just one or at most two cups being consumed in very small sips so that it takes around three to five minutes to drain the cup. The composition of Mariánské Lázně's waters differs markedly from spring to spring and their specific properties and effects are spelled out in detailed notices posted at each source. The Forest Spring (Lesní Pramen) is apparently good for releasing mucus from the nasal passages. Indeed it is described as 'excellent for expectorating'. I think a good number of my fellow hotel guests may have been availing themselves of it, as there was a lot of coughing and spluttering at mealtimes. Somewhat alarmingly, the medical notes go on to say 'it is possible to dissolve kidney stones made of uric acid from the Forest Spring, but we have to be aware that other kidney stones might actually start growing.' The water from the Cross Spring is supposedly beneficial for the gallbladder, liver and for constipation but dangerous for those with high blood pressure. The Rudolph Spring is recommended for older clients, being especially beneficial for osteoporosis; the Caroline Spring has urological benefits; and the Ferdinand Spring is so heavily saline that it has to be treated with great care. Drinking from the Ambrose Spring, whose high iron content is good for anaemia, is supposed to increase sexual potency and desire. It was frequent glasses from this source that supposedly gave Goethe the vigour to pursue his relationship with Ulrike and it is still recommended for people who want to fall in love.

There is still some work to be done to restore the town to its former glory. The former Weimar Hotel where Edward VII stayed is derelict and awaiting restoration. When I peered through a window, an old bath and massage table stood forlornly in the middle of an otherwise deserted ground floor. Neither looked quite old enough, alas, to have been used by Bertie. Other buildings from La Belle Époque have been splendidly and sensitively restored. Perhaps the most impressive are the Nové Lázně, or New Baths, built between 1892 and 1896, which now house the town's most luxurious spa hotel. I tried to book in there for my stay but it was fully occupied by Russians. I did however enjoy a three-hour session in its Roman baths, based on the Gellért Baths in Budapest, which were surprisingly empty. There are two pools, flanked by columns of Salzburg red marble and housed in an imposing hall, together with steam rooms and saunas. Leading off the hall are doors labelled 'Massage', 'Mudpacks' and 'Hydrotherapy'. In an adjoining corridor patients in dressing gowns were sitting waiting for more radical treatments, including gas baths, inhalations and injections, colonic irrigation and various kinds of electro- and magnetic therapy.

On either side of the main entrance to the Nové Lázně hotel are the Imperial and Royal Spa Cabins built for the use of Franz Joseph and Edward VII respectively. A receptionist kindly let me see the former with its magnificent marble columns and terracotta-tiled walls and floor. The latter was out of bounds having been hired by a Russian guest. These two monarchs remain prominent figures in Mariánské Lázně today. Modern statues of both of them, standing in close proximity but not actually facing each other, have been erected in the *Kurpark*, near its entrance from the main street opposite the Hotel Belvedere. A young Franz Joseph is dressed in military uniform, while the English king wears an overcoat and his Homburg hat (Plate 12). A portrait of Edward VII in full state robes greets those going into the first-floor dining room in the Nové Lázně hotel and the hotel library is named after him but there is no mention anywhere of his philandering.

Today's *Kurgäste* seem to have largely forsaken the more hedonistic pastimes and pleasures of their predecessors. The only faint traces of it that I could detect among those staying in my hotel were the large glasses of beer with which most of them accompanied their silent evening meals (which almost invariably involved a meat course served with four or five dumplings) and the plates of cakes and sweets with which they invariably ended them. The other main indulgence are the *oplatky*, or wafers, for which Marienbad was long famous. These are said to have originated from communion wafers, a reminder of the spa's Catholic roots, and resemble ice-cream cones in their consistency. At the height of Marienbad's popularity in 1900s there were twenty-two factories in the town producing four million wafers a year. They are still popular and people can be seen walking round munching them, sometimes as an accompaniment to their sips of water. The beer spa has arrived here although the somewhat desperate marketing – a leaflet shoved into my hand offered a free return taxi trip from Karlovy Vary to the Mariánské Lázně beer spa – suggests that it is perhaps not doing very well. Those taking the cure seem quite content with their daily glass of

Pilsner Urquell and would not, I imagine, relish the prospect of an hour-long soak in a beer-filled bath any more than I did.

The overall impression that modern Mariánské Lázně gives, in common with other European spas today, is of health triumphing over hedonism. This is certainly the approach taken by the town museum which makes a particular feature of having 'a unique collection of rectal and bilious stones'. A display cabinet contains a large stone the size of a duck egg extracted from some unfortunate patient's bladder and a collection of stones weighing more than 460 grammes (1lb) found in a single kidney. Nearby a display of surgical instruments includes 'rectal attachments for enterocleaning', tongs for measuring subcutaneous fat and a rather frightening array of syringes and forceps. The museum occupies what is supposedly the oldest house in the town, where Goethe lodged on his last visit in 1823. There are mock-ups of the rooms in which he stayed, together with a model of him courting Ulrike and poems that he wrote expressing his grief when she rejected him.

Goethe is, indeed, a ubiquitous presence around the town. In front of the museum a bronze statue erected in 1993 replaces one made in 1932 but melted down by the Nazis during the war to make munitions. Another statue erected in 1975 close to the Forest Spring Colonnade shows him standing next to a young lady. A recently published guidebook is at pains to point out that this is not Ulrike, as many people think, but rather his Muse, a purely symbolic character representing the inspirational goddess of poets. A similarly chaste interpretation is provided on a panel fixed to the sandstone obelisk sited near a bench in the woods where he often sat with Ulrike. It makes no mention of his amorous activities when fired up by the aphrodisiacal properties of the Ambrose Spring but rather reproduces a verse from his *Wanderer's Night Songs* in a translation by Henry Wadsworth Longfellow, which speaks of the quiet and restful atmosphere of the woods.

The only slight hint of the old spirit of Marienbad that I could find were notices attached to a birch tree by the main colonnade suggesting that if you kissed someone under its leaves on 1 May, 'you stay fresh for the whole year'. Although I was there on 1 May, I did not see a single soul taking advantage of this invitation. Overall, der Kurschatten, as it has been popularly understood, seems largely to have disappeared in modern Mariánské Lázně. Indeed, the unusual disposition of seats in the Kurpark seems positively to discourage it. As well as traditional park benches, there are a large number of isolated single seats of a kind I have seen nowhere else. Presumably designed for those wishing to sit alone and undisturbed, they encourage the solitary introspection that has been such a prominent occupation of spa-goers through the centuries.

There is one German spa that still makes much of der Kurschatten in its traditional form. The fountain in the main street of Bad Wildungen (see page 10 & Plate 11) is not the only modern reminder of it for today's Kurgäste. A prominent mural in the lobby of one of the main hotels depicts a determined, rather portly wife attempting to restrain her balding husband from joining three shapely ladies standing by the water's edge. Alongside graphic displays of surgical instruments and the tumours, stones and cysts they have removed, a series of historical tableaux in the excellent Quellemuseum feature those who are clearly either the subjects or the objects of Kurschatten, including a young lady avoiding the gaze of an older gentleman at the roulette table and another swooning in bed while a handsome doctor stands over her. The museum has a substantial section devoted to der Kurschatten and even provides copies of a poem on the subject for visitors to take away. The eight-piece Bulgarian Kurorchester does its bit too, playing Fritz Kreisler's Liebesleid, reflecting on the sorrows of a doomed love affair, and 'Strangers in the Night'. It has to be said that there is no hint of scandalous affairs among the middle-aged couples on wellness breaks or the solitary invalids and convalescents browsing in the shops selling Zimmer frames and trusses. Most of the clinics in Bad Wildungen specialise either in urology or in psychosomatic medicine, including hypochondria. For their patients there are darker, more pressing shadows which continue to make spas haunted as well as hidden places.

BIBLIOGRAPHY

Aldous, Richard, *The Lion and the Unicorn* (London: Pimlico, 2007)

Allen, Nick, 'May the Steam Be with You', *Russian Life* 47:1, Jan–Feb 2004

Anderson, Emily (ed.), *The Letters of Beethoven*, 3 vols (London: Macmillan, 1961)

Anstey, Christopher, *The New Bath Guide: Or, Memoirs of the B-r-d Family*, 7th edn (London: J. Dodsley, 1770)

Aronsohn, Eduard, *Erfahrungen und Studien über die Indikationen der Emser Kur* (Berlin: Verlag Ems, 1912)

Austen, Jane, *Northanger Abbey* (London: Folio Society, 1960)

—, *Persuasion* (London: Folio Society, 1961)

Battestin, Martin and Battestin, Ruthe, *Henry Fielding: A Life* (London: Routledge, 1989)

Beard, Mary, *Pompeii: The Life of a Roman Town* (London: Profile Books, 2009)

de Bennetot, Arlette, *Madame de Sévigné aux eaux de Vichy* (Vichy: Compagnie Fermière, 1966)

Bennett-Ruete, Jackie, 'A Social History of Bad Ems: Spa Culture and the Welfare State in Germany' (PhD thesis, University of Warwick, 1987)

Bensusan, S. L., *Some German Spas* (London: Noel Douglas, 1925)

Bergeron, Pierre, *Voyage ès Ardennes en 1619* (Liège: L. Grandmont-Donders, 1875)

le Blanc, Abbé Jean-Bernard, *Lettres d'un François* (Amsterdam, 1751)

Bleymehl-Eiler, Martina, *Der Kurschatten: ein Tabu bei Licht betrachtet* (Bad Schwalbach: Apothekenmuseum, 2007)

Bradley, Ian, 'Taking the Waters', *New Society*, 23 August 1985

—, *Water Music: Music Making in the Spas of Europe and North America* (Oxford: Oxford University Press, 2010)

—, *Water: A Spiritual History* (London: Bloomsbury, 2012)

British Medical Association, *The Spa in Medical Practice* (London: British
   Medical Association, 1951)
Brook-Shepherd, Gordon, *Uncle of Europe: The Social and Diplomatic Life
   of Edward VII* (London: Collins, 1975)
Browne, Thomas, *Works*, ed. Simon Wilkin, Vol. 2 (London: George Bell,
   1888)
Buchan, John, *The House of the Four Winds* (Stroud: Alan Sutton, 1993)
Burman, Lionel, 'The Wedgwoods and the Doctors', *Medical Historian*
   (Bulletin of the Liverpool Medical History Society), No. 13, 2002–2003
Burney, Fanny, *Evelina* (London: Oxford University Press, 1968)
Burr, Thomas, *A History of Tunbridge Wells* (London: M. Hingeston, 1766)
Burton, Robert, *The Anatomy of Melancholy*, 6th edn (New York: Wiley &
   Putnam, 1847)
Cayleff, S., *Wash and Be Healed: The Water-Cure Movement and Women's
   Health* (Philadelphia: Temple University Press, 1987)
Chambers, Thomas, *Drinking the Waters: Creating an American Leisure
   Class at Nineteenth-Century Mineral Springs* (Washington: Smithsonian
   Institute, 2002)
Chapman, R. W., *Jane Austen's Letters* (Oxford: Oxford University Press,
   1952)
Chatwin, Bruce, *Utz* (London: Jonathan Cape, 1988)
Claridge, Richard, *Hydropathy; or The Cold Water Cure, as practiced by Vincent
   Priessnitz* (London: James Madden, 1843)
Cobbett, William, *Rural Rides* (London: Thomas Nelson, 1934)
Croutier, Alev Lytle, *Taking the Waters* (New York: Abbeville, 1992)
Cruse, Audrey, *Roman Medicine* (Stroud: Tempus, 2004)
Cunningham, John (ed.), *400 Years of the Wells* (Tunbridge Wells: Civic
   Society, 2005)
Darwin, Erasmus, *Collected Letters* (Cambridge: Cambridge University
   Press, 2012)
Defoe, Daniel, *A Tour through England and Wales*, Vols 1 & 2 (London: J. M.
   Dent and Sons, 1928)
—, *From London to Land's End* (London: Cassell & Co., 1888)
Deutscher Bäderverband, *Begriffsbestimmungen für Kurorte* (Bonn, 1972)
Dibdin, Charles, *The Musical Tour of Mr Dibdin* (Sheffield, 1788)
Dolan, Brian, *Ladies of the Grand Tour* (London: HarperCollins, 2001)
Dover, Kenneth, *Greek Homosexuality* (London: Duckworth, 1979)
Dostoyevsky, Fyodor, *The Gambler*, trans. C. J. Hogarth (London:
   J. M. Dent and Sons, 1962)

Eidloth, Volkmar (ed.), *Europäische Kurstädte und Modebäder des 19. Jahrhunderts* (Stuttgart: Konrad Theiss Verlag, 2012)

Eliot, George, *Daniel Deronda* (Oxford: Clarendon Press, 1984)

Evans, Edward (ed.), *Tertullian's Homily on Baptism* (London: SPCK, 1964)

Fawcett, Trevor, *Voices of Eighteenth-Century Bath* (Bath: Ruton, 1995)

Fielding, Henry, *The History of Tom Jones*, Vol. 2 (Oxford: Clarendon Press, 1974)

Fisher, John, *Memories of Admiral of the Fleet, Lord Fisher* (London: Hodder & Stoughton, 1919)

Forbes, Elliott (ed.), *Thayer's Life of Beethoven*, Vol. 1 (Princeton: Princeton University Press, 1967)

Ford, Ford Madox, *The Good Soldier* (Oxford: Oxford University Press, 2008)

Garzoni, Tommaso, *La Piazza universale di tutte le professioni del mondo* (Firenze: Olschki, ed., 1996)

Goldsmith, Oliver, *The Life of Richard Nash* (London: Newbery & Frederick, 1762)

Granville, Augustus Bozzi, *Spas of England*, 2 vols (Bath: Adams & Dart, 1971)

—, *The Spas of Germany* (Memphis: General Books, 2012)

Graves, Richard, *The Spiritual Quixote* (London: J. Dodsley, 1792)

Grech, Nikolai, *Pis'ma s dorogi po Germanii* (St Petersburg: Tipografiia N. Grecha, 1843)

Grenier, Lise (ed.), *Villes d'eaux en France* (Paris: Institut Français d'Architecture, 1985)

Hahn, Gernot von, *Wunderbares Wasser* (Aarau: AT Verlag, 1980)

Harcup, John, *The Malvern Water Cure* (Great Malvern: Cappella Archive, 2010)

Headley, Joel, *The Alps and the Rhine* (New York: Wiley & Putnam, 1845)

Hesse, Hermann, 'A Guest at the Spa' in *Autobiographical Writings*, ed. Theodore Ziolkowski, trans. Denver Lindley (New York: Farrar, Straus & Giroux, 1971)

Heywood, Audrey, 'A Trial of the Bath Waters: The Treatment of Lead Poisoning', *Medical History* Supplement No. 10, 1990

Hibbert, Christopher, *The Grand Tour* (London: Weidenfeld & Nicolson, 1969)

Hildesheimer, Wolfgang, *Mozart*, trans. Marion Faber (London: J. M. Dent and Sons, 1985)

Hodder, Edwin, *The Life and Work of the Seventh Earl of Shaftesbury* (London: Cassell & Co., 1892)

Howells, William Dean, *Their Silver Wedding Journey* (eBook, Project Gutenberg, 2006)

Hüfner, Gerhard, *Die Sozialkur* (Kassel: Meister, 1969)

Hunt, Violet, *The Desirable Alien at Home in Germany* (London: Chatto & Windus, 1913)

Hunter, Grace, 'Diary of visit to Red Sulphur Springs, 1838' (http://exhibits.hsl.virginia.edu/springs/redsulphurgracediary/) Accessed 22 January 2020

Jackson, Ralph, *Doctors and Diseases in the Roman Empire* (London: British Museum Publications, 1988)

James, Henry, *Complete Stories 1874–1884* (New York: Library of America, 1999)

—, *Confidence* (London: Macmillan, 1921)

Jenkins, Roy, *Gladstone* (London: Macmillan, 1995)

Jennings, Bernard, *A History of the Wells and Springs of Harrogate* (Harrogate: Borough Council, 1981)

Jones, I. E., 'Growth and Change in Llandrindod Wells since 1868', *Radnorshire Society Transactions* Vol.45, 1975

Kasper, Peter, 'The Future of the Spas' in *Swiss Spas Today* (Bad Ragaz: Verband Schweizer Badekurorte, 1981)

Kneipp, Sebastian, *My Water Cure* (Kempten, Bavaria: Joseph Koesel, 1894)

Langham, Mike and Wells, Colin, *The Baths at Buxton Spa* (Leek: Churnet Valley Books, 2005)

Large, David, *The Grand Spas of Central Europe* (London: Rowman & Littlefield, 2015)

Lennard, Reginald, 'The Watering Places' in *Englishmen at Rest and Play* (Oxford: Clarendon Press, 1931)

Lermontov, Mikhail, *A Hero of Our Time*, trans. J. H. Wisdom and Marr Murray (London: Hodder & Stoughton, 1912)

Lever, Charles, *Arthur O'Leary: His Wanderings and Ponderings* (Boston: Little, Brown, 1894)

de Limbourg, J-P., *New Amusements of the German Spa*, Vol. 2 (London: Davis, 1764)

Mackaman, Douglas Peter, *Leisure Settings: Bourgeois Culture, Medicine and the Spa in Modern France* (Chicago: University of Chicago Press, 1998)

Mallat, Antonin, *Vichy à travers les âges* (Vichy: Imprimerie Centrale Bourbonnaise, 1934)

Mann, Thomas, *Confessions of Felix Krull, Confidence Man*, trans. Denver Lindley (Harmondsworth: Penguin, 1958)

Mansfield, Katherine, *In a German Pension* (New York: Dover Publications, 1995)

Martin, Alfred, 'A Historical Sketch of Balneology', *Medical Life* Vol. 34 No. 5 (New York, 1927)

Martin, Robert, *Tennyson: The Unquiet Heart* (London: Oxford University Press, 1980)

Mattern, Susan, *The Prince of Medicine: Galen in the Roman Empire* (Oxford: Oxford University Press, 2013)

de Maupassant, Guy, *Mont-Oriol*, trans. Marjorie Laurie (New York: Turtle Point Press, n.d.)

—, *Oeuvres complètes*, Vol. XIX (Paris: Louis Conard, 1910)

Meades, Jonathan, 'This Year in Marienbad', *The Times*, 2 January 1988

Mercier, Henry, *Les Amusements des bains de Bade* (Lausanne: Éditions SPES, 1922)

Metcalfe, Richard, *Life of Vincent Priessnitz* (Richmond, Surrey: Metcalfe's London Hydro, 1898)

Mirbeau, Octave, *Les Vingt et un jours d'un neurasthénique* (Paris: Union Générale, 1977)

de Montaigne, Michel, *Essays, travel journal and letters*, trans. Donald Frame (London: Hamish Hamilton, 1958)

Morgan, Benjamin, 'Literary Transmissions and the Fate of a Topic: The Continental Spa in Post-1840 British, Russian and American Writing' (PhD thesis, University College London, 2014)

Moriata, Douglas, *Practical Side of Saratoga Springs As a Health Resort* (Saratoga Springs, 1920)

Morris, Christopher (ed.), *The Illustrated Journeys of Celia Fiennes* (London: MacDonald, 1982)

Morshead, Owen, *Everybody's Pepys* (London: G. Bell & Sons, 1926)

Moryson, Fynes, 'Itinerary', *Retrospective Review* Vol. XI (London: Baldwin, Cradock & Joy, 1825)

Münz, Sigmund, *King Edward VII at Marienbad* (London: Hutchinson, 1934)

de Nerval, Gérard, *Lorely* (Paris: Le Divan, 1928)

Neumann, Dieter and Lehr, Rudolf, *Menschen, Mythen, Monarchen in Bad Ischl* (Bad Ischl: Tourismusverband, 2008)

Osborne, Bruce and Weaver, Cora, *Aquae Britannia: Rediscovering 17th-Century Springs and Spas – In the Footsteps of Celia Fiennes* (Malvern: Cora Weaver, 1996)

—, *Aquae Malvernensis: The Springs and Fountains of the Malvern Hills* (Malvern: Cora Weaver, 1994)

Peeters, Luc and Houbrechts, David, *Spa: Ville Thermale* (Brussels: Prisme Editions, 2016)

Penrose, John, *Letters from Bath* (Gloucester: Alan Sutton, 1983)

Pepys, Samuel, *Diary: A Selection* (London: Penguin Books, 2003)

Phillips, E. D., *Greek Medicine* (London: Thames & Hudson, 1973)

Piranomonte, Marina, *The Baths of Caracalla* (Milan: Electa, 2006)

Pope, Alexander, *Works*, Vol. VI (London: Longman, Brown & Co., 1847)

Porter, Roy (ed.), *The Medical History of Waters and Spas* (London: Wellcome Institute, 1990)

—, 'Consumption: Disease of the Consumer Society?' in *Consumption and the World of Goods*, eds John Brewer and Roy Porter (London: Routledge, 1993)

Porter, Roy and Rousseau, George, *Gout: The Patrician Malady* (New Haven: Yale University Press, 1998)

Punch magazine, 11 September 1858

Purbeck, Jane and Purbeck, Elizabeth, *Neville Castle*, Vol. 1 (London: Dutton & Cawthorn, 1802)

Rapp, Christian and Rapp-Wimberger, Nadia, *Bad Ischl* (Vienna: Christian Brandstätter Verlag, 2016)

Rattue, James, *The Living Stream: Holy Wells in Historical Context* (Woodbridge: Boydell Press, 2001)

Ridley, Jane, *Bertie: A Life of Edward VII* (London: Chatto & Windus, 2012)

Rolls, Roger, *Diseased, Douched and Doctored: Thermal Springs, Spa Doctors and Rheumatic Diseases* (London: London Publishing Partnership, 2012)

Rotherham, Ian, *Spas and Spa Visiting* (London: Shire Publications, 2014)

Rubovszky, András, *Hotel Gellért* (Budapest: Széchenyi Publishing House, 1988)

Rumbold, Horace, *Recollections of a Diplomatist*, Vol. 1 (London: Edward Arnold, 1902)

Schapiro, Leonard, *Turgenev: His Life and Times* (Oxford: Oxford University Press, 1978)

Schretzenmayr, A., 'Kur, Kurarzt und Kurklinik', *Münchener Medizinische Wochenschrift* No. 11, 1965

Sebald, W. G., *Austerlitz*, trans. Anthea Bell (London: Hamish Hamilton, 2001)

de Seingalt, Jacques Casanova, *Memoirs*, trans. Arthur Machen, Vol. 6 (London: privately printed, 1894)

Seneca, Lucius Annaeus, *Epistulae Morales ad Lucilium*, trans. Richard Gummere (London: Loeb Classical Library, 1917)

Shepherd, William, *The Life of Poggio Bracciolini* (Liverpool: Harris Brothers, 1837)

Silliman, Benjamin, *A Journal of Travels in England, Holland & Scotland* (New York: Ezra Sargeant, 1810)

Smollett, Tobias, *The Expedition of Humphry Clinker* (Athens: University of Georgia Press, 1990)

Stevenson, William, *A Successful Method of Treating the Gout by Blistering* (Bath: Cruttwell, 1779)

Stott, Anne, *Wilberforce: Family and Friends* (Oxford: Oxford University Press, 2012)

Strachan, Michael, *The Life and Adventures of Thomas Coryate* (Oxford: Oxford University Press, 1962)

Strouse, Jean, *Alice James: A Biography* (London: Jonathan Cape, 1981)

Swafford, Jan, *Johannes Brahms: A Biography* (London: Macmillan, 1998)

Tennyson, Alfred, *Letters*, eds Cecil Lang and Edgar Shannon, Vol. 1 (Oxford: Clarendon Press, 1982)

Terrier, J. C., 'Remarks on Balneotherapy' in *Swiss Spas Today* (Bad Ragaz: Verband Schweizer Badekurorte, 1981)

Thomson, William, *Spas that Heal* (London: A. & C. Black, 1978)

Tolstoy, Leo, *Anna Karenina*, trans. Aylmer and Louise Maude (Oxford: Oxford University Press, 1958)

Trollope, Anthony, *Can You Forgive Her?* (London: Trollope Society, 1989)

—, *The Small House at Allington* (London: Trollope Society, 1997)

Turgenev, Ivan, *Smoke,* trans. Constance Garnett (London: Heinemann, 1906)

Twain, Mark, *A Tramp Abroad* (New York: Oxford University Press, 1996)

D'Urfey, Thomas, *The Bath: Or, The Western Lass: A Comedy* (London: Peter Buck, 1701)

Vauthey, Max, *Vichy et Napoléon III* (Vichy: Éditions Shave, 1984)

Vida, Mária, *Spas in Hungary in Ancient Times and Today* (Budapest: Semmelweis Kiadó, 1992)

Vieth, David M. (ed.), *The Complete Poems of John Wilmot, Earl of Rochester* (New Haven: Yale University Press, 1968)

Wagner, Richard, *My Life* (London: Constable, 1911)

Warner, Richard, *Bath Characters* (London: G. Wilkie & J. Robinson, 1807)

Wechsberg, Joseph, *The Lost World of the Great Spas* (New York: Harper Row, 1979)

Wesley, John, *Primitive Physic* (Boston: Cyrus Stone, 1858)

Wheen, Francis, *Karl Marx* (London: Fourth Estate, 1999)

White, Giles, *Hot Bath: The Story of the Spa* (Bath: Nutbourne Publishing, 2003)

Wilson, John, *CB: A Life of Sir Henry Campbell-Bannerman* (London: Constable, 1973)

Wood, Ellen, *East Lynne* (Oxford: Oxford University Press, 2008)

Yegül, Fikret, *Bathing in the Roman World* (Cambridge: Cambridge University Press, 2010)

Yeo, Isaac Burney, *The Therapeutics of Mineral Springs and Climates* (London: Cassell & Co., 1904)

Zeldin, Theodore, *France 1848–1945* Vol. 2 (Oxford: Oxford University Press, 1977)

INDEX